Pharmacology for Anaesthetis

For Churchill Livingstone:

Publisher: Geoffrey Nuttall
Project Editor: Lowri Daniels
Copy Editor: Teresa Brady
Production Controller: Mark Sanderson
Sales Promotion Executive: Caroline Boyd

Pharmacology for Anaesthetists

Noel Cass MB BS FRCA FANZCA
Formerly Professional Associate in Anaesthesia;
Formerly Examiner in Pharmacology, ANZ College of Anaesthesia;
Examiner to Australasian College of Emergency Medicine,
University of Singapore and National University of Malaysia;
Nuffield Prizewinner

Linda Cass MB BS FANZCA
Renton Prizewinner

CHURCHILL LIVINGSTONE
EDINBURGH LONDON MADRID MELBOURNE NEW YORK AND TOKYO 1994

CHURCHILL LIVINGSTONE
Medical Division of Longman Group UK Limited

Distributed in the United States of America by
Churchill Livingstone Inc., 650 Avenue of the Americas,
New York, N.Y. 10011, and by associated companies,
branches and representatives throughout the world.

First published 1994

ISBN 0-443-04639-5

British Library Cataloguing in Publication Data
A catalogue record for this book is available from the British Library.

Library of Congress Cataloging in Publication Data
Cass, Noel.
  Pharmacology for anaesthetists / Noel Cass, Linda Cass.
    p.   cm.
  Includes index.
  ISBN 0-443-04639-5
  1. Pharmacology. 2. Anesthesiology. I. Cass, Linda. II. Title.
  [DNLM: 1. Pharmacology. 2. Anesthetics. QV 81 C343p 1994]
RD82.C37   1994
615'.1--dc20
DNLM/DLC
for Library of Congress   93-7322
                                                                              CIP

The
publisher's
policy is to use
paper manufactured
from sustainable forests

Produced by Longman Publishers Singapore Pte Ltd
Printed in Singapore

Contents

Preface

Anaesthetists must be able not only to understand and apply a knowledge of pharmacology, but also, at some stage, demonstrate this knowledge in examinations. This book evolved from demands for a text that fulfils this role. Three previous editions of the fore-runner of this book, *Pharmacology Notes*, have been published by the Australian and New Zealand College of Anaesthetists (ANZCA). Based on lecture-tutorials given in the basic medical science course for the ANZCA, these notes have served as a basis for examination preparation and revision for practising anaesthetists over many years.

Topics of importance in clinical anaesthesia and examinations have been addressed. For clarity, diagrams and tables frequently accompany the text. The presented data have been accumulated from a number of standard texts and publications. In some instances an approximate value has been given where sources vary. Clearly, fuller discussions of some topics will be found in reference literature.

Chapter 22 has been included to emphasise the importance of developing a satisfactory examination technique, to recall and set out knowledge. This chapter comprises a skeleton answer to a general pharmacology question, followed by answers to nine typical styles of question set in the written examination.

Acknowledgements and thanks are due to many colleagues who, (knowingly or unknowingly), have helped to clarify and criticise many aspects of the text; and to the ANZCA for encouragement and access to past examination papers and reports.

1993   L.C.
                                                                         N.C

1. Pharmacokinetics

1.1 ADMINISTRATION

The proportion of a drug given orally which reaches the general circulation is the **bioavailability** of that drug. It is reduced by:

1. inactivation in the gut: e.g. tetracyclines are chelated
2. poor absorption: neostigmine
3. partial metabolism by enzymes in the gut mucosa: chlorpromazine
4. metabolism by the liver – the **first-pass effect** – before the portal venousblood joins the vena cava: nifedipine.

The *percentage absorption* can be measured by

$$\frac{\text{area of the plasma level–time curve (oral)} \times 100}{\text{area of the plasma level–time curve (i.v.)}}$$

ORAL

Necessary conditions

A low and predictable first-pass effect: e.g. antihistamines. Minimal absorption is desirable if the effects are to be confined to the gut: e.g. neomycin.

Rate of absorption

Dependent on Fick's Law: concentration gradient, membrane area and permeability. The **amount absorbed** is also dependent on the length of time of exposure of the drug to the gut (see note on digoxin and metoclopramide below).

1. A weak acid, e.g. aspirin, is poorly ionized in the presence of gastric acid, and is more lipid-soluble. It is thus rapidly absorbed from the stomach.

2. Rapid absorption occurs from the small gut as its surface area is so great, hence a rapid passage from the stomach is desirable. **Metoclopramide** (Maxolon) enhances gastric emptying and increases the rate of absorption.

Note. 1. Some drugs (digoxin) are poorly soluble: a rapid transit through the intestine due to metoclopramide may not allow full absorption.

1

Conversely, drugs which decrease intestinal motility (tricyclics, disopyramide) enhance the absorption of digoxin.

2. Gastroenteritis may also shorten transit time and may result in the failure of an oral contraceptive or a reduced effect of digoxin.

Time of onset

This relates to the rate of absorption, and is very variable, depending on the contents and motility of the stomach.

Emptying of the stomach is delayed when there is:

1. intestinal atony due to obstruction or peritonitis
2. labour, especially if obstructed
3. trauma, e.g. fractures, head injury
4. emotional stress, e.g. awaiting anaesthesia and surgery
5. opioid premedication
6. pain

The rate of absorption is also influenced by the preparation of the drug. Absorption rate falls in this order: solutions, suspensions, capsules, tablets, enteric-coated tablets, slow-release preparations.

Advantages

The oral route is simple and preferred to injection. For this reason non-opioid analgesics are being increasingly exploited.

Disadvantages

1. Drugs may *damage the gut*: aspirin.
2. They may be *destroyed by secretions*: esters and gastric acid.
Note. A drug may be protected by a film soluble only in alkali, enabling it to pass the stomach and be absorbed in the small gut. **Slow-release drugs** are dissolved in poorly-soluble vehicles e.g. resins. As gut secretions dissolve the vehicle, the drug is available for absorption. Slow release prolongs the duration of action and avoids the risk of a high peak in plasma level. Some antihistamines can be given in this way as they are effective in low concentrations in the plasma.
3. *Monoamine oxidase* (MAO) in the gut wall may inactivate drugs e.g. tyramine (in aged cheese, yeast). MAO inhibitors suppress this protective function, and tyramine can then produce a *hypertensive crisis* by releasing noradrenaline.
4. *Hyperosmolar solutions* e.g. sweet drinks stay in the stomach until diluted, with an increased risk of vomiting during induction if anaesthesia is begun too soon after they are imbibed.
5. Absorption is *unpredictable*.

SUBCUTANEOUS

Necessary conditions

1. The drug and its solvent must not cause pain or irritation: ketamine, extravenous thiopentone.

2. It must have a reasonably prolonged action or it may be eliminated as quickly as it is absorbed. Extravenous neuromuscular blockers have little measurable effect in moderate doses.

Rate of absorption

Slow, due to the low perfusion: 0.05 ml blood/ml tissue per minute. Blood loss or hypothermia depresses skin circulation, slowing absorption further. The classical example is subcutaneous morphine injection in hypovolaemic shock: repeated injections are given because of the lack of response. With resuscitation, the circulation returns and all the drug is quickly absorbed, giving the effects of overdose. To avoid this problem, drugs are given intravenously, diluted if necessary, and slowly until the response is obtained. Hyaluronidase hastens absorption by decreasing the viscosity of the ground substance of connective tissue, allowing wider diffusion and greater exposure to capillary beds.

Delay in absorption may be achieved by:

1. implanting a solid pellet of the drug, e.g. steroid
2. dissolving the drug in oil, e.g. penicillin
3. converting a soluble drug into an insoluble salt, e.g. atropine mucate
4. addition of adrenaline 0.001% (1 : 100 000 or 10 µg/ml).

Advantages

Slow absorption achieves a low concentration for a longer time, even if the drug is being eliminated, e.g. soluble insulin is far more effective subcutaneously than given as a bolus intravenously (i.v.) (but it can be given as an infusion).

Time of onset

Effects appear within 30 minutes and reach their maximum in 1 hour, but great variation is found.

INTRAMUSCULAR

a. Usually less painful than subcutaneous route.

b. Absorption depends on perfusion, resting muscle having 2 ml blood/100 ml muscle per minute compared with subcutaneous tissue, 1 ml/100 ml per minute. In the neonate intramuscular (i.m.) suxamethonium in dosage of 3 mg/kg produces paralysis in about 3 minutes. However drugs which are poorly soluble in water at physiological pH may be absorbed very slowly: e.g. diazepam, digoxin. This is an advantage with procaine penicillin and ultralente insulin.

c.
Muscle is less prone to chemical injury and infection than subcutaneous fat.

INTRAVENOUS

This is the most rapid way of distributing a drug widely.

Note. Due to the blood–brain barrier ionized drugs do not normally enter the central nervous system (CNS). This is an advantage with neuromuscular blocking drugs (which have profound effects if injected into the cerebrospinal fluid CSF) but a disadvantage with many antibiotics which must be given intrathecally to treat meningitis.

Necessary conditions

1. A suitable vein must be accessible. The technique of venipuncture must be learned and practised.

2. The drug must be soluble in water or some suitable vehicle: e.g. propofol in soya bean oil, egg phosphatide and glycerol; diazepam in propylene glycol or soya bean oil/water emulsion (Diazemuls) or in bile acid/lecithin/water emulsion (Mixed Micelles).

3. The injection should not injure veins. Aseptic phlebothrombosis takes some days to appear but may persist for weeks; it may make the dorsal hand veins unpleasantly tender, and occurs occasionally after injection of thiopentone and other hypnotics. Many drugs, e.g. pethidine, tubocurarine, release histamine which causes reddening and sometimes a wheal over the vein, but this resolves within 1 hour.

Advantages

1. The effect may be seen in one circulation time, e.g. thiopentone. The required dose is thus easily found, with additional injections if necessary. If onset is slower, e.g. 2–3 minutes with non-depolarizing neuromuscular blockers, a dose based on body weight is used, e.g. vecuronium 0.09 mg/kg.

2. Elimination occurs in proportion to the plasma level and is therefore enhanced. Radio-opaque dyes excreted by the kidney enable intravenous pyelography to be performed.

3. Drugs which damage tissues in high concentration, e.g. many cytotoxics, are rapidly diluted by blood: injections into the femoral vein are diluted tenfold before they reach the carotid arteries.

Disadvantages

1. Venipuncture may be difficult in oligaemic shock, in patients who are nervous, cold or obese, in advanced rheumatoid arthritis and in infants aged 3–18 months.

2. Injection outside the vein (due to part or all of the needle bevel being outside the vein) may injure nearby tissues. Thiopentone causes local inflammation and soreness, but the dose–effect relationship is still obscure.

3. Accidental injection into an aberrant artery or one lying adjacent to a vein may cause spasm or thrombosis with thiopentone. This is a chemical irritation and not related to alkalinity, as an equally alkaline solution of sodium carbonate is without effect.

4. Rapid injection produces a very high peak concentration, with the risk of acute toxicity. With thiopentone a brief period of hypotension is common, and apnoea may occur. With **aminophylline**, caution must be taken to avoid the risk of hypotension and sudden death: the dose of 5–8 mg/kg must be diluted and given over 20 minutes.

When peripheral circulation is slow due to *depleted circulating volume* or *peripheral venous stasis* as in cardiac failure, an injection of 3–5 mg/kg of thiopentone produces a much higher peak plasma concentration than usually occurs, and profound depression of the circulation may result. A *smaller dose* should be chosen and given slowly: dilution to 1% may help to assess the minimum adequate dose while avoiding side-effects.

INFUSION

For many drugs whose action needs to be prolonged, a steady plasma level within fairly narrow limits is optimal, as this avoids the risk of undesirable effects from too high a level or a waning of effect from too low a level. For example, morphine may cause respiratory depression with overdose, or pain may recur if the level falls.

Note. Regular high peaks of bactericidal antibiotics may be more effective in destroying the microorganisms at the time of cell division.

Infusions of the shorter-acting neuromuscular blocking drugs and hypnotics are also useful. As it takes 5 half-lives to reach a steady concentration of an infused drug, it is necessary to inject a **loading dose** before the infusion is begun. Figures 1.1.1 and 1.1.2 illustrate this important principle.

Loading dose = desired concentration × volume of distribution (Vd)

For morphine, whose desired concentration is 65–80 nanogram/ml and Vd is 3.2 litre/kg (l/kg), the loading dose in a 15 kg child would be:

$$\frac{15 \times 3200 \times 65}{1\,000\,000} \text{ mg}$$

$$= 3 \text{ mg}$$

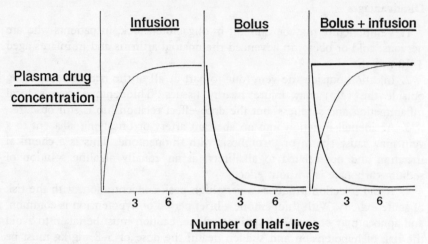

Fig. 1.1.1 Bolus and infusion: this combination achieves the desired steady plasma level of drug, as opposed to repeated bolus doses.

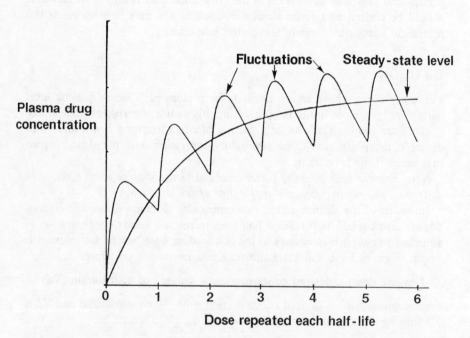

Fig. 1.1.2 Repeated bolus doses: a steady plasma level is reached only after 5–6 half-lives, and the fluctuations may reach a toxic level during the rises or an ineffective level during the falls. With morphine this may be manifest as undue depression followed by return of pain before the next injection.

This dose can also be calculated from the usual recommendation of 0.1–0.2 mg/kg.

The **infusion rate** can be calculated either from the *half-life* (which is the time taken for the plasma level to fall 50%) or the *elimination rate*, which measures the volume cleared of the drug each minute. The *half-life* of morphine is about 3 hours (3 h). In the 15 kg child above, the infusion would be set to deliver up to 1.5 mg every 3 h: the range would be delivered by diluting 0.5 mg/kg in 50 ml of 5% dextrose and infusing 1–5 ml/h (10–50 $\mu g \, kg^{-1} \, h^{-1}$) depending on the response.

The **elimination rate** of morphine is 15 ml $kg^{-1} \, min^{-1}$ (15 ml/kg per minute). The dose per minute would thus be:

$$\frac{15 \text{ ml} \times \text{loading dose (3000 } \mu g)}{Vd \, (3200 \text{ ml} \times 15 \text{ kg})}$$

which is about 1 $\mu g \, kg^{-1} \, min^{-1}$, the upper range as calculated from the half-life. In clinical practice with a depressant drug like morphine, it is clearly desirable to start at a low rate and increase it if necessary, with repeated observations for respiratory depression.

Special considerations for drug infusions

1. Need for an i.v. infusion with a *one-way valve* above the drug entry point to avoid reflux into the line if the cannula blocks, and sudden overdose if the cannula then clears. Alternatively, a dedicated i.v. line is optimal (preferably near a central vein if a short-acting drug, e.g. nitroprusside, is being given). *Note*. The subcutaneous route may be adequate if the drug is not irritating and has a long half-life.

2. An *infusion syringe or drip-controller*.

3. *Adequate instructions* for staff.

INHALATION

This route is of special interest to anaesthetists and its kinetics must be understood. It has often been overlooked by candidates in examinations.

Necessary conditions

1. Adequate depth and rate of respiration (*minute volume of respiration*). It is important to remember that opioid analgesics and most intravenous induction agents are respiratory depressants. Most inhalation agents are themselves respiratory depressants, especially in the higher concentrations used for induction. A moderate overdose can readily produce severe respiratory acidosis: a mild rise in end-tidal carbon dioxide (to about 50 mmHg) is commonly seen during spontaneous respiration with inhalation anaesthesia.

2. *Normal blood and gas distribution in the lungs.* In lobar collapse due to a foreign body, neoplasm or a mucus plug, gas access may be totally prevented. In severe emphysema both gas mixing and lung perfusion are abnormal. When the lung *FRC (functional residual capacity = residual + expiratory reserve volumes) falls below the critical closing volume during expiration* (this occurs after 40 years of age), *patchy atelectasis occurs.* The consequent impaired ventilation/perfusion ratio may be partially compensated by increasing the concentration of oxygen and the anaesthetic vapour inhaled.

3. *Adequate normal alveolar surface* (90 square metres in an adult). Lung collapse (due to pleural effusion, subdiaphragmatic pressure or bronchial obstruction) or emphysema reduces the effective area. Diffusion through the alveolar cells is also impaired by oedema fluid (alveolar-capillary block).

4. A means of *regulating the inspired concentration* of the vapour accurately.

5. *Avoidance of increased deadspace*, especially from inappropriate breathing equipment or inadequate fresh gas flow.

Advantages

1. Rapid and effective blood level is obtained.
2. Excretion occurs mainly by the lungs and is not impaired by metabolic or renal disturbance.
3. Anaesthetic vapours and gases do not injure the pulmonary epithelium, although ciliary activity is depressed.

Disadvantages

Higher vapour concentrations may be irritant and cause breath-holding during induction. Ether vapour provokes bronchial secretions which are inhibited by atropine.

Other points of importance

The tension of the gas in mixed venous blood depends on:

1. The *solubility of gas in blood* (blood–gas partition coefficient).
2. The *solubility of the gas in the tissues, and their blood supply.* From these can be found the amount of gas needed to saturate the tissues at the necessary concentration, and how long this will take.
3. The *duration of the anaesthetic.* As this lengthens, the vapour pressure of the agent in the tissues approaches that in the arterial blood. Ultimately, at saturation, the venous blood vapour tension equals that in arterial blood, but this takes some hours; with vapours that are very soluble in fat (e.g. halothane), it takes days.

Recovery from an inhaled agent

This will depend on:

1. Its *solubility in fat and muscle*. If this is high, excretion will take longer, especially after a long anaesthetic when the vapour pressure in the fat has come closer to equilibrium with that of the CNS.

2. The *proportion of the blood which is cleared of the vapour by the lungs* with each passage of the blood. If the ratio of alveolar ventilation to cardiac output is 4:5 (the V/Q ratio is 0.8), the proportion removed is:

nitrous oxide: 63%   enflurane: 30%   halothane: 26%   isoflurane: 36%

The proportion falls as the solubility partition coefficient rises, but with a very fat-soluble agent like halothane the vapour is also being rapidly redistributed into the fat at the end of a short anaesthetic and recovery is quicker than would be predicted by pulmonary elimination.

3. The *respiratory deadspace*. If this is increased, e.g. by a facemask, elimination is slowed.

4. *Rebreathing* of exhaled gases, as may occur with an oxygen mask with inadequate fresh gas flow.

INTRATHECAL

Local anaesthetics are given by this route to obtain controlled and intense block with limited dosage, e.g. saddle block requires only 1.5 ml 5% lignocaine (75 mg).

Note

1. Scrupulous asepsis must be practised as the CSF has minimal cellular defences against infection, and immune antibodies cannot enter unless the blood–brain barrier is damaged.

2. Local anaesthetics become 'fixed' in nerve tissue, limiting their diffusion, e.g. lignocaine no longer diffuses after 5 min. *Systemic absorption* rate from the subarachnoid space is variable. For lignocaine the absorption follows first-order kinetics with a half-life ($t\frac{1}{2}$) of about 70 min; for bupivacaine 30% is absorbed quickly in about 50 min, the remainder slowly (about 400 min).

3. Loss of CSF through dural puncture may cause severe headache, and even symptoms of meningitis (vomiting, photophobia). An epidural injection of the patient's blood (blood patch) may improve this dramatically but may leave local fibrosis which makes subsequent epidural instrumentation less reliable.

Drugs which do not pass the blood–brain barrier must be injected intrathecally, e.g. streptomycin.

EPIDURAL

The epidural space is an annulus between the bony vertebral canal and the spinal cord and meninges. It is small opposite the cervical expansion (vertebra C5, 1.0–1.5 mm) and lumbar expansion (vertebra L2, 5–6 mm) of the cord. It contains venous plexuses and fat. The former pose a risk of unintended intravenous injection of local anaesthetics or analgesics, and the latter competes with nerve tissues for lipophilic drugs. Spread in the space occurs widely, and may become intracranial even though the spinal dura is fused with the periosteum at the foramen magnum, apparently limiting the space anatomically. Absorption from the epidural space occurs partly through the dura, and extradural morphine has been associated with respiratory depression. Drugs are ultimately removed by absorption into blood vessels. The latter can be slowed by adding adrenaline 1:100 000 to local anaesthetic solutions.

Some typical kinetics: **Morphine:** peak plasma concentration at about 8 min; fraction crossing the dura, 1–5%; peak CSF morphine occurs between 0.5 and 1.5 h; CSF clearance is very slow (0.15–0.45 ml/min). **Lignocaine:** absorption is biphasic, rapid initially then slow (Ionescu et al 1989).

SURFACE APPLICATION

Skin

Absorption is slow, but special preparations are effective. **EMLA cream** (Eutectic Mixture of Local Anaesthetics) contains lignocaine and prilocaine bases and is applied under an occlusive dressing, producing skin analgesia in an hour. **Scopolamine**, in a vehicle of mineral oil and polyisobutylene, may be applied to the skin behind the ears (a predictable site for absorption) for motion sickness. It is reported to last 3 days. Clonidine and fentanyl have also been given transdermally. The phosphonium insecticides (malathion, sarin) are readily absorbed from skin or conjunctiva, and poisoning can result. Gases and vapours diffuse slowly through skin.

Mucosal surfaces

1. Eyes

Solutions must be nearly isotonic. Local anaesthetics, adrenaline, analogues of atropine, physostigmine and antibiotics are commonly used. Absorption is rapid, unless the drugs are highly ionized, e.g. neostigmine.

Note. Excess drug solution flowing down the nasolacrimal duct is swallowed. The consequent absorption of atropine from 1% drops (0.6 mg/drop) may cause toxicity (delirium, hyperthermia).

2. Mouth

Sublingual absorption avoids entry through the portal system and first-pass metabolism. **Nitroglycerine** (Trinitrin) for angina is well established. **Buprenorphine,** a partial opioid agonist, has 55% bioavailability. Onset is slow. A high hepatic clearance ensures safety if the tablet is swallowed. **Morphine** is also absorbed, but its unpleasant taste limits its use.

3. Nose

Adrenaline-like decongestants, antihistamines and antidiuretic hormone are well absorbed. Drug abusers use this route for cocaine: the resulting vasoconstriction may cause ischaemic necrosis.

4. Trachea and bronchi

Absorption of local anaesthetics is reported to be slow in rate but large in amount (Satoh 1988). Hence dosage should be limited, e.g. lignocaine, 4 mg/kg. **Beta-adrenergic agonists** e.g. salbutamol, terbutaline are used by aerosol for asthma.

5. Rectum

Absorption is slow, necessitating a high concentration and hence a large dose with a drug such as thiopentone. Paracetamol, 15 mg/kg, and diazepam 0.5 mg/kg are effective.

FURTHER READING

Ionescu T I, Drost R H, Winckers E K A et al 1989 Epidural morphine for abdominal aortic surgery: pharmacokinetics. Regional Anesthesia 14:107–114
Satoh Y 1988 Pharmacokinetics of lidocaine and monoethylglycine-xylidide after the intratracheal administration of lidocaine. Japanese Journal of Anesthesiology. 37: 1192–1198

1.2 DISTRIBUTION OF DRUGS

On entering the circulation, drugs are distributed to:
   1. The extracellular fluid of the blood (plasma): about 3 litres (3 l) or 4% of body weight.
Examples are albumin and plasma expanders which cannot enter red cells or escape either through or between vascular endothelial cells. *Plasma protein binding* confines a fraction of many drugs to plasma: the bound fraction has no effect on tissues. Binding is *reversible*: the drug concentration in the plasma falls as drug enters the tissues, and more bound drug then becomes free and can enter the tissues. Thiopentone is highly bound: 77% at pH 7.8.

This accounts for its solubility in blood as it is poorly soluble in water at pH 7.4.

2. The total extracellular fluid (interstitial + plasma): 18 l, or 25% of body weight.

Highly ionized or *polar* drugs: neuromuscular (NM) blockers are good examples. They leave the capillaries by passing between the endothelial cells. *Exceptions* are ions for which there are special transport mechanisms: sodium, potassium.

3. The whole body water: 50 l or 70% of body weight; e.g. glucose, urea, ethyl alcohol.

Note: Urea enters the CSF slowly, enabling it to decrease intracranial pressure by osmotically transferring water to the plasma. Equilibration between CSF and blood may later give a rebound rise.

4. Specific sites of distribution: e.g. iodine and the thyroid gland.

Acceptors are tissues which bind drugs without any pharmacological response, as opposed to *receptors*, which produce pharmacodynamic responses. Acidic mucopolysaccharides act as acceptors to curare-like drugs, reducing the free fraction available for NM block.

The blood–brain barrier is a permeability barrier between the blood and the CNS. It is composed of vascular endothelium and adjacent astrocyte foot processes with tight intercellular junctions which make it behave like an epithelial membrane: drugs must be lipid-soluble to enter the brain. The CSF differs from brain tissue by being more accessible: the choroid plexus capillaries are fenestrated and more permeable. In the *neonate and in a number of pathological states* (cerebral embolism, post-convulsions, trauma, radiation injury, anaemia, hypoxia, hypertensive crisis, cerebral tumours and meningitis), the barrier is less effective. It is also reduced in some areas: e.g. the area postrema in the floor of the IVth ventricle where morphine enters and affects the chemoreceptor trigger zone. *Levodopa* passes the barrier and is converted to dopamine (which is deficient in the corpus striatum in Parkinson's disease). Carbidopa does not cross the barrier, but inhibits conversion of levodopa to dopamine outside the CNS; smaller doses of levodopa are then effective, and its systemic side-effects reduced.

An example of **selective entry** of a lipophilic drug is seen with propranolol whose brain–plasma ratio is 26:1. It may cause hallucinations, but the related beta-adrenoreceptor blocking drug, atenolol, is not lipophilic (its ratio is 1:5) and it has no CNS effects.

TISSUE PERFUSION

The rate of rise of drug concentration in a tissue depends on the **perfusion** and the **tissue–blood partition coefficient.** The latter expresses the relative solubility in blood and tissue at 37°C. Table 1.2.1 shows the different levels of perfusion for the various tissues. Figure 1.2.1 represents this graphically. Table 1.2.2 shows changes in cardiac output and in tissue perfusion during

Table 1.2.1 Tissue perfusion rates in a 70 kg patient

Tissue	Perfusion (per minute)			Tissue mass (kg)	% Body weight	Oxygen uptake	
	ml blood/ ml tissue	litres blood	% Cardiac output			ml/min	%
Lungs	4.80	5.00	100	0.90	1.2		
Liver	1.00	1.50	25	1.5–1.80	2.5	51	20
Kidneys	4.90	1.30	25	0.30	0.4	20	7
Brain	0.54	0.80	15	1.20–1.50	2.0	63	23
Heart	0.70	0.22	4	0.33	0.5	23	9
Muscle							
Rest	0.02	0.90	17	30	40–50	55	20
Exercise	1.00	35.00	80	30	40–50	2700	90
Skin	0.06	0.25–0.45	6	5	7.0	11	5
Bone							
Marrow	0.13	0.2	4	1.50	2.5		
Fat	0.01	0.1	2	7–12	10–20		

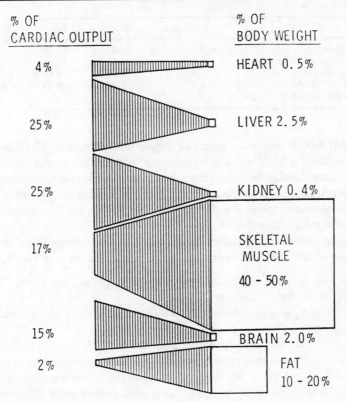

Fig. 1.2.1 Perfusion and tissue mass.

anaesthesia, reported in animal studies, and Table 1.2.3 shows the perfusion of various tissues according to their grouping (vessel-rich, vessel-poor, muscle, fat). The rich perfusion of the brain and heart accounts for the rapid and profound effect of drugs such as thiopentone and inhaled anaesthetics.

Table 1.2.2 Cardiac output and its distribution: changes during anaesthesia. These data are reported in animal studies. (Note: increased tissue perfusion can compensate for a fall in cardiac output.)

Drug	Cardiac output	Perfusion
Ketamine (1.2 mg/kg)	20% decrease	Brain 100% increase Muscle 40% decrease
Halothane (1.5 MAC, minimum anaesthetic alveolar concentration)	25% decrease	Heart 30% decrease Muscle 60% decrease Kidney 50% increase Liver 50% increase
Enflurane (1.5 MAC)	Unchanged	Brain 25% increase Liver 30% increase Heart 30% decrease Muscle 65% decrease

Table 1.2.3 Perfusion in various tissue groups. Vessel-poor groups include bone, ligament, tendon and cartilage

	Vessel-rich	Muscle	Fat	Vessel-poor
% Body mass	9.0	50.0	19.00	22.00
Volume (litres in 70 kg man)	6.0	33.0	14.50	12.50
% Cardiac output	75.0	18.0	5.40	1.50
Perfusion in litres/min, when cardiac output = 6 l/min	4.5	1.1	0.32	0.07

Redistribution is also a result of *differential perfusion*. The vessel-rich tissues achieve a high initial concentration of drug, but as the plasma level falls the drug diffuses back into the blood. The vessel-poor tissues have a low initial level, and continue to absorb the drug: their *rising concentration of drug is achieved mainly from the falling concentration in the vessel-rich tissues*. Hence the term *redistribution*.

After an injection of thiopentone given over 20 seconds there are three processes which initially lower the plasma concentration (see Fig. 1.2.2.):

a. *Venous mixing* distributes the drug throughout the blood. This is complete after about 4 minutes.

b. During a., *a rapid transfer* of drug occurs *into the extracellular fluid compartment*.

c. *Entry into the intracellular fluid;* the rate depends on the tissue perfusion. CNS equilibrates very quickly, producing unconsciousness, but a. and b. lead to an early fall in drug concentration, and awakening occurs. Muscle tissue concentration equilibrates with plasma after 20 minutes, a perceptible time after awakening. Fat equilibrates with plasma after about 40 minutes.

The process of elimination then results in a slow and protracted fall in plasma level which continues for about 12 h, during which time there is a feeling of mild sleepiness and impairment of concentration. With methohexitone this

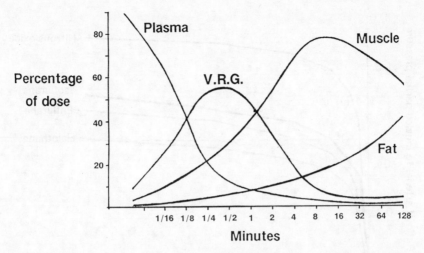

Fig. 1.2.2   Thiopentone redistribution (partly diagrammatic). V.R.G. – vessel-rich group of tissues.

period is shorter, and with the now-discarded propanidid, an ester of eugenol, very rapid recovery was due to chemical hydrolysis.

BLOOD–GAS EQUILIBRATION OF INHALATIONAL ANAESTHETICS (See Fig. 1.2.3)

The blood and tissue solubility significantly alter the rate at which equilibration is reached: with particularly soluble anaesthetic vapours, the following is seen:

1. A slower induction: equilibration between the vapour pressures in arterial blood and tissues may take hours to achieve. This is due to the agents being soluble in muscle and, especially, fat. These tissues comprise 50% of the body weight but receive only 20% of cardiac output: a large bucket and a small hose. In contrast the CNS is 2% of body weight with 15% of cardiac output – a small bucket and a fire-hose. In addition, the relatively lower solubility of the anaesthetic in blood must be taken into account, further delaying equilibrium.

2. A longer time to reach a steady state (vapour pressure equal in blood and tissues).

3. Prolonged excretion: a slower recovery. It can be seen that a fall in vapour pressure of the anaesthetic in blood will result in a corresponding fall in the CNS, but that the fall in fat will be much slower. This may lead to a slow recovery of consciousness after prolonged deep anaesthesia as the drug coming from the fat will continue to affect the CNS because only a fraction of the vapour is excreted with each passage through the lungs.

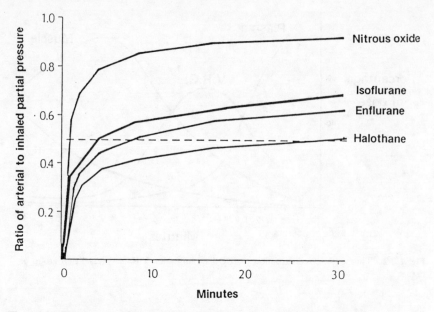

Fig. 1.2.3 Blood/gas equilibration. The rapid initial rise represents equilibration between the alveoli and inspired vapour. The 'knee' of the curve represents the saturation of blood, and the plateau the slow equilibration of the tissues.

An important factor in pulmonary clearance of vapours is the *blood–gas partition coefficient*. If this is high (that is, the drug is very soluble in blood) only a small fraction will be exhaled as the blood passes through the lungs. This is because a small amount leaving the blood will raise the partial pressure of the vapour in the alveoli into equilibrium with the vapour pressure of the agent dissolved in the blood. For example, if the ventilation/ perfusion ratio is normal (4 litres/5 litres or 0.8), and there is no rebreathing, *26% of halothane (partition coefficient 2.3) is removed during one pulmonary circulation*. With *nitrous oxide (coefficient 0.47), 63% is removed*.

Table 1.2.4 illustrates this concept, comparing nitrous oxide and halothane. The equilibration half-times of various tissue groups are shown. Note that

Table 1.2.4 Uptake of inhalation anaesthetic: effect of increased alveolar ventilation or reduced cardiac output. The equilibration times in minutes of various tissue groups are shown

	Partition coefficient	Lung/blood	Vessel-rich group	Muscle	Fat
Nitrous oxide	0.47	1.0	3.6	42	108
Alveolar ventilation × 2		0.4	2.6	38	103
Cardiac output × 0.5		0.8	5.2	76	204
Halothane	2.30	14.7	20.4	206	2330
Alveolar ventilation × 2		3.8	10.2	158	2140
Cardiac output × 0.5		7.7	20.4	315	4280

Table 1.2.5   Inhalation agents: MAC (minimum anaesthetic alveolar concentration) solubilities and pulmonary clearance

Agent	MAC %	Blood–gas partition coefficient at 37°C	Oil–water partition coefficient at 37°C	% Cleared from blood at each passage through lung
Enflurane	1.68	1.9	120	30
Halothane	0.74	2.3	220	26
Isoflurane	1.15	1.4	120	36
Nitrous oxide	105.00	0.47	3.2	63
Trichlorethylene	0.17	9.15	400	8
Nitrogen	–	0.014	5.2	98
Oxygen	–	0.023		97

Notes:
1. MAC falls by 1% with each 1% increase in nitrous oxide (N_2O) concentration. With 70% N_2O, isoflurane MAC is 0.5%.
2. MAC falls by 10% with morphine 0.2 mg/kg.
3. Gases diffuse slowly through the skin. After 100 minutes of inhalation with 70% N_2O, 3.6 ml/min per square metre
4. Note the very high clearance of nitrogen. A useful aid is the 3,4,5 rule: after 3 minutes breathing 4 litres fresh gas flow in a circle with absorber, expired gas contains less than 5% of nitrogen.
5. The percentage cleared with each passage of blood through the lungs is given by:

$$\frac{1 \times 100}{1 + 1.2 \times (\text{Blood/gas}) \text{ solubility}}$$

alveolar ventilation and cardiac output also interplay, affecting equilibration half-times. Table 1.2.5 further details blood–gas partition coefficients and pulmonary clearances of various inhalational anaesthetics, nitrogen and oxygen.

Note. Halothane has an extremely high fat/blood solubility (about 100) which results in an *apparent exception* to the above. The fat stores become saturated very slowly. After a short anaesthetic (up to 30 minutes), when the halothane is turned off, halothane is redistributed to fat stores as well as being exhaled. These two processes result in a faster recovery from anaesthesia than would be expected from the solubility of halothane in blood and other tissues. A further factor is metabolism which eliminates up to 20% of halothane, contrasting with enflurane (2–8%) and isoflurane (0.2%).

It will be appreciated from the above discussion that the physical characteristics of inhalational agents influence their kinetics. Table 1.2.6 gives a more complete outline of physical data. These data are of greater relevance when considering administration (viz. vaporization) of volatile agents. It is included at this point to facilitate memory.

PLACENTAL TRANSFER (See Table 1.2.7)

Gases, sedatives, narcotic analgesics, local and general anaesthetics cross the placenta by simple diffusion. The area of exchange is 11 m², the thickness 3.5 μm.

Table 1.2.6   Inhalation anaesthetics: physical data

Drug	Boiling point, °C	Vapour pressure, mmHg	Saturated vapour, at 20°C	Specific gravity of liquid, at 20°C	ml vapour/ml liquid at 20°C
Enflurane	56	175	23%	1.52	198
Halothane	50	241	32%	1.87	227
Isoflurane	48	252	33%	1.52	196
Nitrous oxide	– 88	39000	gas		
Diethylether	35	443	58%	0.72	233

Table 1.2.7   Factors influencing placental transfer

Drug	Ionization
	Lipid solubility
	Plasma protein and red cell binding
	Concentration gradient
	Molecular weight
	Metabolites
	Tissue binding
Maternal	Blood volume
	Uteroplacental blood-flow
	Uterine contractions
	Normality of placenta
Fetal	Fetal liver
	Shunting in the fetal circulation
	Immaturity of the brain.
	Fetal plasma, red cells and pH
	Compression of umbilical cord.

Pethidine: fetal level reaches 77% of maternal and persists for over 2 h.

Thiopentone: fetal level rises rapidly, equilibrating with maternal in 2–5 min.

Tranquillizers: benzodiazepines cross readily, and also enter breast milk.

Atropine: crosses rapidly.

Neuromuscular blockers: being highly polar, do not cross readily, but small amounts have been found in the fetus. With alcuronium a fetal–maternal gradient of 0.26 was found, but no effect on the fetus was detected. Suxamethonium is not destroyed by the placenta. The small amount transferred has been found to affect a neonate who was homozygous for dibucaine-resistant pseudocholinesterase.

Local anaesthetics: Transfer occurs, and fetal bradycardia has been noted after bupivacaine. More profound fetal effects led to the abandonment of mepivacaine (Carbocaine): this agent is poorly metabolized by the fetus in contrast to lignocaine and bupivacaine.

Placental circulation

For placental transfer to occur, the utero-placental circulation must be normal. This is disturbed during labour or placental insufficiency, leading to erratic and unpredictable drug transfer. There is good evidence that the state of the baby at delivery is affected more by the adequacy of the uteroplacental circulation than by drugs given to the mother.

Fetal circulation

The majority of umbilical venous blood goes to the ductus venosus, bypassing the portal vein and liver. Hence the first-pass effect is negligible. The fetal liver is also immature, making the fetus dependent on the maternal route for drug elimination.

Plasma protein binding (PPB) in pregnancy

This falls, increasing the unbound (diffusable) fraction of drugs such as lignocaine, diazepam and pethidine. PPB in the fetus also differs from that of the mother, and may result in a different intensity of effect.

PHARMACOKINETIC MODELS

The distribution of a drug depends on its solubility in water and lipids, and its capacity to bind to special sites. The body may be represented by *compartments*, which the drug enters and leaves at specified *rate constants*. If the drug is freely diffusible throughout the body, e.g. ethyl alcohol, a one-compartment model applies (see Fig. 1.2.4).

Ionized (polar) drugs are soluble in water but not lipids. They exchange between the plasma (central compartment) and interstitial fluid (peripheral compartment): a two-compartment open model (see Fig. 1.2.5).

When a drug enters cells or crosses the blood–brain barrier or becomes fixed to special sites, further compartments and rate constants enter the picture, and kinetics become correspondingly complex.

EQUATIONS DESCRIBING KINETICS

Some symbols and equations are commonly used.

Vd is the *volume of distribution*, and is related to the amount of drug in the body and its plasma concentration.

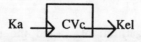

Fig. 1.2.4   One-compartment model. Vc = volume of central compartment; C = concentration of drug in central compartment; CVc = amount of drug in central compartment; Ka = rate constant of absorption; Kel = rate constant of elimination; (excretion and metabolism).

Central compartment   **Peripheral compartment**

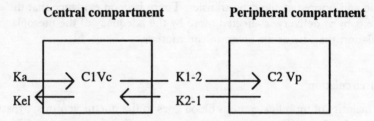

Fig. 1.2.5 Two-compartment open model. Vc = volume of central compartment; Vp = volume of peripheral compartment; Ka = rate of absorption into, and Kel = rate of elimination from, central compartment; C_1, C_2 = concentrations of drug in central and peripheral compartments, respectively; C_1Vc = amount of drug in central compartment; C_2Vp = amount of drug in peripheral compartment K_{1-2}, K_{2-1} = rate constants for transfer between central and peripheral compartments.

Hence:

$$Ab = Vd \times Cp$$

where Ab is the amount of drug and Cp the plasma concentration.

β is the *elimination rate*, and

$$Vd = \frac{dose}{\beta \times \text{area under the plasma concentration–time curve}}$$

(The plasma concentration–time curve is shown in Fig 1.2.6)

An **approximation of the Vd** *(the apparent volume of distribution)* is also given by:

$$Vd = \frac{dose}{Cp_o}$$

(Cp_o is the value of the linear plasma concentration curve during elimination extrapolated back to the time of injection: time zero).

Clearance, **Cl**, is the volume of blood or plasma cleared of drug each minute, and is expressed as:

$$Cl = \beta \times Vd$$

The *plasma half-life*, $t\frac{1}{2}\beta$, also called the *elimination half-life*, is expressed as:

$$t\frac{1}{2}\beta = \frac{0.693 \times Vd}{Cl}$$

0.693 is the natural logarithm of 2, and the formula is based on the exponential fall in plasma concentration with first-order kinetics. In zero-order kinetics the fall is linear (e.g. the metabolism of ethyl alcohol), and the concept of half-life is unnecessary.

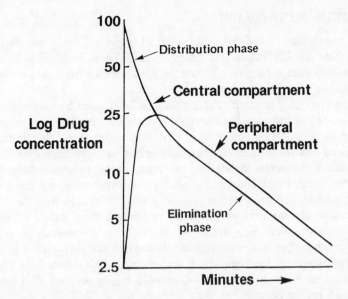

Fig. 1.2.6 Two-compartment mode: a representation of the drug concentrations in the central and peripheral compartments following a bolus intravenous injection.

With multiple doses of a drug with a long half-life, a steady state will ultimately ensue, with elimination equalling dosage (see Fig. 1.2.2).

The *volume of distribution in the steady state* (**Vdss**)

$$= \frac{\text{Total quantity of drug in the body}}{\text{Plasma concentration in the steady state (Cpss)}}$$

Vdss is used in calculating infusion rates and the elimination half-life.

The *plasma concentration in the steady state*, **Cpss**, is expressed as:

$$\text{Cpss} = \frac{F \times D}{Cl \times T}$$

where F is the fraction of the dose reaching the central compartment (100% with i.v. dosage), D is the dose and T the time between doses. It can also be expressed as:

$$\text{Cpss} = \frac{t\frac{1}{2}\beta \times F \times D}{0.693 \times \text{Vdss} \times T}$$

This relationship is used in determining infusion rates.

FURTHER READING

Eger II E I 1974 Anesthetic uptake and action. Williams and Wilkins, Baltimore

1.3   DRUG METABOLISM

Drug metabolism is used to describe all types of drug transformation. Metabolism usually inactivates drugs, hence the term *'detoxification'*, but many metabolites are active: e.g. succinylmonocholine from suxamethonium, and salicylic acid from aspirin.

Metabolites may be toxic. Paracetamol is inactivated by conjugation with glucuronide and sulphate, but a small amount is converted by liver microsomal oxidase to a reactive intermediate alkylating metabolite. This is normally conjugated and inactivated by glutathione, but in overdosage glutathione is depleted and the metabolite injures liver cells, leading to hepatic failure in 4–6 days. Prophylaxis with glutathione precursors (cysteamine, methionine) prevents toxicity when paracetamol reaches a toxic level (250 µg/ml).

Metabolic change may be necessary to make a drug active: digoxin and thyroxine are called 'pro-drugs'. At birth, drug metabolism is not fully developed: hence neonates are resistant to digoxin and thyroxine. Conversely, they are susceptible to drugs which are inactivated by metabolism: chloramphenicol dosage is reduced to one-quarter (25 mg/kg per day). At 5 weeks the dose is 75 mg/kg per day.

Antipyrine is a model drug for liver metabolism as it is not plasma protein-bound and enters hepatocytes freely, and it is entirely hydroxylated and not excreted unchanged. Hence its rate of elimination measures the metabolic capacity of the liver.

Elimination half-life ($t\frac{1}{2}\beta$) of a drug is the time taken for its plasma concentration to fall 50%. Most drugs are eliminated at a rate proportional to their concentration (first-order kinetics), their concentration falling exponentially (Fig. 1.3.1). If the concentration on the Y-axis is plotted logarithmically, a straight line represents the fall in plasma level (Fig. 1.3.2).

Some drugs are metabolized at a constant rate irrespective of their concentration, displaying **zero-order kinetics.** Ethyl alcohol is metabolized at a rate of about 10 ml/h in a 70 kg person. Others, e.g. phenytoin when given in overdose, saturate the metabolic processes and decay linearly for a time, and then exponentially when metabolic pathways are no longer saturated.

Distribution/redistribution kinetics must be differentiated from metabolism: α represents the stage of distribution after rapid i.v. injection. The plasma concentration falls due to dilution in the total plasma volume, and distribution to the extracellular fluid and richly perfused tissues. Thiopentone undergoes a rapid fall in plasma level ($t\frac{1}{2}\alpha$ = 5 min) after administration, but its elimination $t\frac{1}{2}\beta$ is 8–10 h. Hence the early arousal is followed by a prolonged mild soporific effect.

METABOLIC CHANGES

Phase 1 pathways generally inactivate drugs by hydrolysis, oxidation or reduction, but with pro-drugs may activate them. *Phase 2* pathways involve conjugation with highly polar molecules.

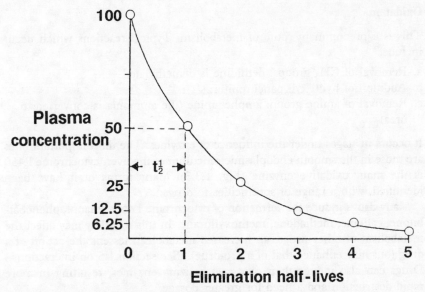

Fig. 1.3.1   Elimination. First-order kinetics: linear plot.

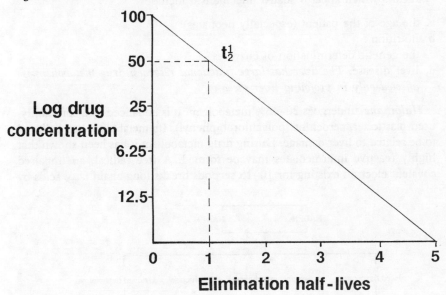

Fig. 1.3.2   Elimination. Semi-logarithmic plot.

Hydrolysis

An enzymatic breakdown involving water. Esters are split into an alcohol and an acid (usually organic). Acetylcholine breaks into choline and acetic acid, suxamethonium into two molecules of choline and succinic acid (via succinylmonocholine: the enzyme is plasma cholinesterase).

Oxidation

This is a predominant route of metabolism. Typical reactions which occur include:

a. Removal of CH_3 groups: pethidine is demethylated
b. Addition of hydroxyl: pancuronium
c. Removal of amine group: amphetamine (the ammonia is converted to urea)

It occurs in stages under the influence of enzymes. The most important ones are those in the smooth endoplasmic reticulum of the liver: cytochrome P450 is the main oxidative enzyme (Fig. 1.3.3). Many forms of it have been identified, with a range of specificities to drugs.

Many drugs induce the formation of cytochrome P450: ethanol, phenobarbitone, caffeine, methadone, methoxyflurane. In this way they may affect the metabolism of other drugs: an increased metabolism lessens the action of a drug (but may enhance that of a pro-drug). (See section 1.5 on interactions.) Drugs can also induce their own metabolizing enzymes, resulting in more rapid destruction and a need for greater dosage.

Factors which affect oxidative metabolism include

a. the age of the patient (especially neonates)
b. nutrition
c. the genetic determination of enzymes
d. liver disease. *The liver has large functional reserves: drug metabolism is affected only in profound liver disease.*

Halothane undergoes 20–46% metabolism. It is enhanced by a commonly-used plasticizer, aerochlor (polychlorobiphenyl). Its metabolites are believed to be related to liver damage. During drug metabolism it has been shown that highly reactive intermediates may be formed. A free radical, an unpaired covalent electron existing for 10–15 seconds breaks long-chain fatty acids by

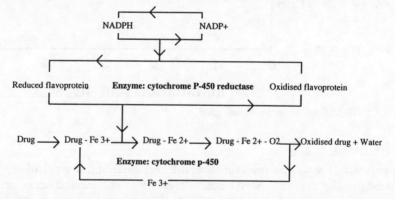

Fig. 1.3.3 The oxidative pathway. (NADPH – nicotinamide–adenine dinucleotide phosphate, reduced form; $NADP^+$ – oxidized form.)

lipid peroxidation, causing centrilobular liver injury. Glutathione absorbs free radicals, protecting against the injury.

Reduction

An intermediate step in metabolism: chloral hydrate (a pro-drug) is reduced to trichlorethanol, a long-acting hypnotic which is later oxidized.

A reductive intermediate occurs in the metabolism of *halothane* in hypoxic conditions (and possibly also when normal oxygenation is maintained). It is hepatotoxic and may account for the halothane hepatitis.

Conjugation

A molecule is added to the drug, converting it from high lipid-solubility to water-solubility, promoting its renal excretion.
Examples:

a. Glucuronic acid: morphine, paracetamol
b. Sulphate: some catechols
c. Acetylation: hydrallazine
d. Methylation: histamine, serotonin.

THE LIVER

All drugs absorbed through the portal system pass through the liver. Many are metabolized (*the first-pass effect*) before reaching the systemic circulation. In cirrhosis the oral bioavailability of pethidine rises from 56% (in normal patients) to over 80%. At rest, 25% of cardiac output flows to the liver, continually exposing drugs to hepatic metabolism. The liver *extracts* a varying proportion of drugs from its blood flow: lignocaine and morphine have a high extraction ratio, paracetamol an intermediate one and diazepam a low one. *Hepatic clearance* depends mainly on blood flow when drugs have a high extraction ratio; but blood flow is less important when drugs are highly protein-bound and readily metabolized.

Effects of liver disease (See Table 1.3.1)

1. Volume of distribution is altered
2. Metabolism may be impaired
3. Plasma protein binding is reduced
4. Extraction of drugs falls as liver blood flow falls. This can be a more important factor than the impaired metabolism, but plasma protein binding is also important.

Note:

1. *The liver has a high exposure to drugs which may injure it.* (See Table 1.3.1)

Table 1.3.1 Half-lives (t½) of drugs in patients with cirrhosis

	% Extraction rate	% Plasma-protein binding	% Change in t½
Highly-extracted drugs			
Lignocaine	83	60–75	+ 300
Morphine	50–75	35	+ 25
Propanolol	60–80	93	+ 300
Verapamil		90	+ 500
Poorly-extracted drugs			
Diazepam	3	99	+ 230
Lorazepam	3	92	+ 35
Theophylline	9	60	+ 450

2. *Some hepatotoxins are dose-related.* (See Table 1.3.2.)
3. *Other hepatotoxins, such as halothane, are unpredictable.* (See Table 1.3.3.)

With halothane, injury is not dose-related, is rare, recurs with further exposure and there may be signs of hypersensitivity (fever, eosinophilia, skin rash). Children are less likely to be affected.

Selective enzyme inhibitors such as monoamine oxidase (MAO) inhibitors (tranylcypromine, iproniazid) have drawn attention to the hazards raised by interfering with drug metabolism. The target organ is the CNS, but MAO in gut epithelium is also affected, permitting absorption of tyramine, and consequent sympathetic overactivity.

There are also non-selective enzyme inhibitors, but they are not used clinically.

Table 1.3.2 Dose-related hepatotoxins

Injury	Drugs
Fatty degeneration	Tetracyclines, salicylates, carbon tetrachloride
Fibrosis, cirrhosis	Methotrexate
Cholestasis	Anabolic steroids, azathioprine
Hepatitis	Isoniazid, salicylates
Angiosarcoma	Vinylchloride monomer

Table 1.3.3 Unpredictable hepatotoxins

Injury	Drugs
Hepatitis	Halothane, phenylbutazone, sulphonamides
Cholestasis	Chlorpromazine, chlorpropamide, erythromycin, oral contraceptives
Chronic hepatitis	Alpha-methyldopa
Granuloma	Hydrallazine, phenylbutazone

1.4   EXCRETION

The lungs and kidneys are the principal routes of excretion, although some metabolites are excreted in bile (e.g. alcuronium). Saliva, sweat and alimentary secretions are minor routes.

LUNGS

Although anaesthetic vapours are excreted predominantly by the lungs, it should be remembered that metabolism does occur to a variable degree.

The *rate at which a gas or vapour is removed depends on:*

1. The *alveolar ventilation*, which depends on the rate and depth of respiration. Tidal volume is particularly important as the physiological deadspace becomes proportionately more as the tidal volume decreases. At higher respiratory rates the tidal volume must decrease, making respiration less efficient: hypercarbia (and hypoxia if inspired oxygen is not increased) will tend to occur.

2. The *solubility of the vapour in the blood* (the blood–gas partition coefficient). If this is high, a small amount of vapour diffusing into the alveolus will raise the vapour pressure into equilibrium with that in the blood, and a small proportion only will be excreted with each passage of blood through the lungs (see Table 1.2.5). Hence recovery will be slower than from vapours with a low coefficient.

3. Factors resulting in *ventilation–perfusion mismatch* in the lung:

i.   Airways obstruction: asthma, neoplasm, foreign body, external pressure (e.g aneurysm)
ii. Reduced alveolar surface: emphysema
iii. Mechanical factors: muscle weakness or partial residual paralysis, obesity, increased abdominal pressure
iv. Central respiratory depression: opiates, deep anaesthesia
v.   Vascular shunting. The normal V/Q is 0.8. It is decreased by atelectasis, lobar collapse and postural changes imposed by surgery and anaesthesia.

KIDNEYS

In a 70 kg man about 1.35 l of blood flow through the kidneys each minute, of which 135 ml are filtered by the glomeruli. Both volumes are decreased in deep anaesthesia. Molecules with a size less than 70 000 daltons are filtered: all anaesthetic drugs are in this category. Many are partly bound to plasma protein, and the *free fraction* only is filtered: this affects the elimination of a drug like pancuronium which is 87% bound. This is not important with lipid-soluble drugs that are entirely reabsorbed by the tubular epithelium, such as thiopentone (77% bound).

The renal tubules reabsorb 99% of the filtrate together with any filtered lipid-soluble drugs. Polar drugs (ionized ones with high water-solubility) are not reabsorbed unless there is a special transport mechanism e.g. sodium ions. Some drugs are actively excreted by the tubules e.g. penicillin. With this drug the rate can be greatly reduced by giving probenecid which competes with other acidic drugs for transport across the cell. For the same reason, probenecid reduces the tubular reabsorption of uric acid.

Assuming that the glomerular filtration rate is 135 ml/min, and that the extracellular fluid is 18 l; and that the drug is confined to this compartment, is not plasma protein-bound and not reabsorbed, the plasma half-life is given by the formula:

$$t_{1/2} = \frac{\log_e 2 \times \text{volume of distribution}}{\text{renal clearance}}$$

$$= \frac{0.693 \times 18000}{135} \text{ i.e. approximately 90 min}$$

Under these conditions only 12% of the drug will remain after 4.5 h, but this time will increase with protein binding, tubular reabsorption or reduced renal blood flow. In anuria, drugs which rely almost entirely on renal excretion must be given with great care, e.g. alcuronium, digoxin; and muscle relaxants which are metabolized, e.g. vecuronium, atracurium, suxamethonium, are preferable.

Tubular excretion is not affected by plasma protein binding as the drug is actively excreted (instead of being filtered in solution). This lowers the unbound fraction and some of the bound drug is freed to restore equilibrium. More of the free drug can then enter the tubular cells and undergo excretion. Conversely, glomerular filtration removes both water and the free drug so the concentration in the plasma is unaltered, and none of the bound drug becomes available for filtration.

Tubular reabsorption of acidic and basic drugs is affected by urine pH. Pethidine is a base: only 4% is excreted (as pethidine or norpethidine) in alkaline urine. Urine may be acidified by 2 g ammonium chloride or 10 g arginine given 6-hourly, leading to greatly increased excretion (22% of a dose as pethidine and 24% as norpethidine). Acidic drugs e.g. salicylic acid are excreted more rapidly in alkaline urine. The mechanism in each case is the reduction of lipid solubility by promoting ionization.

Renal function is immature at birth. Adult values of glomerular filtration are reached at 3–5 months, and of renal tubular capacity at 7 months.

ELIMINATION KINETICS

Glomerular filtration tends to follow first-order kinetics: the amount filtered is proportional to the concentration of free (filterable) drug in the blood.

Renal tubular absorption and excretion are subject to a maximum rate, above which the rate of exchange across the tubular cells is unchanged, following zero-order kinetics.

Renal excretion kinetics are dependent on the drug available in the blood (which together with the extracellular fluid usually comprises the 'central compartment'). If the drug enters the cells or becomes bound to tissues, a multicompartment model applies, and the rate of renal excretion will be affected by the rate at which the other compartments return the drug to the blood.

In the lung, diffusion of anaesthetic vapour to the alveoli follows first-order kinetics, but the overriding factors in excretion are the alveolar ventilation, solubility of the vapour in blood and tissues, and tissue perfusion parameters.

1.5 DOSAGE IN CHILDREN, ADULTS, AND PREGNANCY

Dosage has been related to surface area (as is basal metabolic rate). (*Note:* surface area neonate 0.25 m^2, 2 years 0.5 m^2, 9 years 1.0 m^2, adult 1.73 m^2.) However, dosage based on weight is simple and effective in practice. A safe working rule for paediatric practice is to multiply the adult dose by the child's weight divided by 50. Table 1.5.1 gives a more precise relationship. Up to 10 years a child's weight can be estimated at *twice the age plus 9 kg.* The recorded weight should be checked against this to avoid inadvertent overdosage.

NEONATES AND CHILDREN

Distribution

Total body water is 85% of body weight in the premature infant, 70% in the neonate and 55% in the adult. The increased proportion is mainly in the extracellular fluid: drugs distributed to this space (polar drugs such as muscle relaxants) tend to have a higher dosage requirement/kg. *Note:* neonates are sensitive to non-depolarizing blockers, thus compensating for this effect, but from 1–10 years it is demonstrable.

Table 1.5.1 Dosage and age

		% of adult dose	
	Weight, kg	Related to surface area	Related to weight
Adult	70	100	100
12 years	40	75	57
7 years	23	50	33
1 year	11	25	14
4 weeks	4.5	15	6.4

Blood volume is 90–100 ml/kg at birth, 75 ml/kg at 6 months and 70 ml/kg at 3 years.

Fetal albumin binds drugs less than that of adults: a lower dose of highly protein-bound drugs e.g. thiopentone is required.

Metabolism

Oxidation and glucuronidation are decreased: diazepam has a prolonged half-life (t½). From 1–10 years liver microsomal oxidation is faster than adults, requiring an increased dosage of anticonvulsants compared with adults.

Renal excretion

Excretory capacity is reduced at birth, prolonging the effects of polar drugs e.g. atropine, muscle relaxants. At 6–12 months it reaches adult values.

ADULTS

Dosage is usually based on weight, but this will be erroneous when using a polar drug e.g. muscle relaxant in an obese patient because their proportion of lean tissue mass (muscle) is reduced. It is common to give a 'standard' dose to adults: one ampoule or one tablet. Where precision of dosage is not hazardous e.g. atropine or sedatives, this does not matter. In anaesthesia however dosage should be related to the patient's weight to avoid over- or underdosage. For polar drugs the proportion of lean body mass should also be noted. Anaesthetists should bear in mind the individual variation of response and be prepared to titrate doses until the desired effect is achieved.

OLD AGE

Changes after about 55 years of age tend to reduce dosage (Table 1.5.2).

   a. *Metabolic rate* falls.

   b. *Intracellular water* decreases 0.6%/year, reducing the volume of distribution of drugs which enter cells e.g. thiopentone.

   c. *The bronchial tree, lung tissue and chest wall are less elastic,* increasing the work of breathing. The supine CV (closing volume) falls to the FRC (residual volume plus expiratory reserve volume) at 45 years, resulting in atelectasis with shunting, especially with spontaneous respiration during anaesthesia. At 75 years vital capacity has fallen to 60% of that at 30 years, maximum voluntary respiration to 50% and oxygen uptake to 40%. Pa_{O_2} falls, approximating to the formula:

$$Pa_{O_2} = 104 - (\text{age}/4)$$

1. Inhaled oxygen concentration should be increased.

Table 1.5.2 Changes in old age

Change	Effect
Reduced body water Reduced proportion of muscle Increased proportion of fat	Higher concentration in body fluids
Reduced lung function	Slower uptake and excretion of inhaled agents Prone to respiratory acidosis and hypoxia
Reduced liver function and blood flow	First-pass effect, extraction and metabolism are reduced
Reduced renal blood flow and glomerular filtration rate (GFR)	Slower renal extraction
Blood volume and cardiac output fall	Delayed onset of action: i.v. injections give higher blood levels
Reduced plasma protein	Free fraction of protein-bound drugs rises, enhancing effects

2. Induction will be slower unless inspired concentration of anaesthetic vapour is increased.
3. Recovery from inhalation anaesthesia will be slower.
4. Respiratory acidosis occurs more readily during spontaneous respiration.

d. *Reduced muscle mass* relative to body weight alters tissue compartment volumes e.g. less thiopentone redistribution to muscle occurs.

e. *The size of the liver decreases*, from 2.5% of adult body weight at 30 years to 1.6% at 90 years. Liver blood flow falls, with less drug extraction and metabolism. First-pass effect is reduced.

f. *Renal plasma flow falls*: at 75 years it is 50% of that at 30 years. The number of glomeruli falls. Renal function at 90 years is 50% of that at 30 years. Renal excretion of drugs falls, especially those removed by glomerular filtration e.g. atropine, muscle relaxants.

g. *Cardiac output falls* 1%/year: at 70 years it is 70% of that at 30 years. Blood volume falls: at 70 years it is also 70% of that at 30 years. These changes result in a smaller dose achieving an adequate blood level.

Note: Slowed circulation, reduced blood volume, reduced cardiac output and reduced muscle mass readily lead to overdosage with thiopentone because the anaesthetist continues to inject the drug while waiting for the patient to fall asleep.

h. *Plasma albumin decreases*, especially if there is poor nutrition or blood loss. Protein binding falls: pethidine is 75% bound at 25 years, 35% bound at 75 years. The greater free fraction increases the effect of the calculated dose.

i. *The cerebral cortex* loses 10^3 cells every day: 2×10^7 by 60 years, but there remain 99.98% of the 10^{12} cells present at childhood. Even this loss results in an increased susceptibility to central depressants e.g. opiates, especially in patients with cerebrovascular disease.

j. *Atherosclerosis* reduces perfusions of some tissues (e.g. lower limbs) so that a higher proportion of cardiac output goes to well-perfused tissues (brain, heart).

PREGNANCY

1. *Extracellular and blood volumes* increase.
2. *Plasma protein* concentration falls, with a higher proportion of free drug available e.g. lignocaine, diazepam, pethidine.
3. *Gastric emptying* is slowed.
4. *Glomerular filtration rate* rises, enhancing the excretion of polar drugs.
5. The *placenta* metabolizes some drugs but the effect of this on drugs used in anaesthesia is uncertain.
6. The *functional residual capacity* of the lung falls due to subdiaphragmatic pressure.
7. The *epidural space* is decreased by venous enlargement due to raised intra-abdominal pressure.
8. The *nerves* are more readily blocked by local anaesthetics.
9. *Plasma level of cholinesterase* falls postpartum, but the related increased duration of suxamethonium is usually associated with a heterozygous genotype (E1u E1a).

Drugs in labour and the fetus

Drugs cross the placenta by diffusion down a concentration gradient. Only the free fraction diffuses: the fetal–maternal ratio for bupivacaine is 0.25. The majority of umbilical venous blood goes to the ductus venosus, bypassing the portal vein and liver: there is *negligible first-pass effect*. The fetal liver is immature so that the fetus is largely dependent on the mother for drug elimination. This dependence is of course lost at birth, and drugs given during labour may cause prolonged effects in the newborn. For example *pethidine* has a $t\frac{1}{2}\beta$ of 23 h in the newborn compared with 3–5 h in the mother.

Oxytocin crosses the placenta. Its antidiuretic effects on the fetus may result in hyponatraemia. It also results in reduced uteroplacental blood flow secondary to uterine contractions, which may in turn cause fetal distress seen on cardiotocography.

Beta$_2$-adrenergic drugs are used to inhibit uterine contractions. If continued for 24 h, the baby may be born with hyperinsulinaemia and rebound hypoglycaemia.

Diazepam, previously used to control fitting in pre-eclampsia, causes hypotonia and impaired thermoregulation in the neonate.

2. Pharmacodynamics

Drugs related to anaesthesia act predominantly:

a. *on receptors*
b. *on the cell membrane,* altering the behaviour of ion channels
c. *indirectly,* by acting on enzymes e.g. anticholinesterases prolong the duration of action of choline esters.

DRUGS AND RECEPTORS

Receptors can be identified as chemical groupings on the cell membrane. Large numbers of these are known, with specificity for transmitters and drugs related to them.

The transmitter may be:

1. blocked (ACh and non-depolarizing relaxant)
2. mimicked (ACh and suxamethonium)
3. depleted (noradrenaline and reserpine).

A drug which acts on a receptor to produce a response is termed an *agonist.* If the drug cannot produce a maximum response it is termed a *partial agonist.* A partial agonist displays both agonist and antagonist activity. If given in low dosage with a small dose of a full agonist, the activity of the two is additive. When given with a maximum effective dose of the agonist, it acts as an antagonist, preventing the agonist from achieving its full effect. Morphine is an agonist in producing analgesia, buprenorphine and pentazocine are partial agonists. When given with an agonist, they become antagonists.

Affinity refers to the dosage needed to produce 50% of the maximum response: a lower dosage implies a higher affinity. *Intrinsic affinity* (also called *efficacy*) is a measure of the maximum response the drug can produce.

Potency is a term used in comparing the effective doses of two drugs e.g. halothane with MAC 0.74 is more potent than enflurane (MAC 1.68).

The dose-response curve tends to be non-lincar (see Fig. 2.1). A more useful plot is the *log dose–response curve* (see Fig. 2.2) as the points then fall close to a straight line except for the extremes (which can also be made linear by using a probit plot).

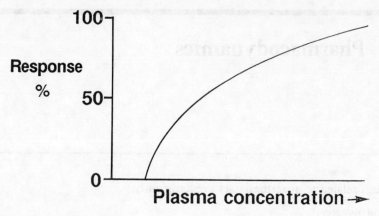

Fig. 2.1 Dose–response curve.

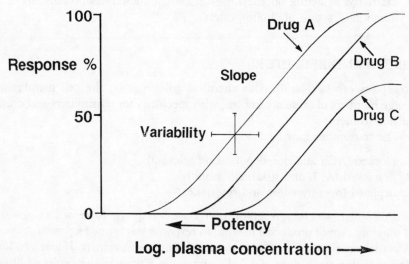

Fig. 2.2 Log dose–response curve. Drug A has a higher affinity than drug B. Drug C is a partial agonist.

Competitive antagonism

In the presence of a competitive antagonist, a full response can be obtained by increasing the dose of the agonist: the log dose–response curve is shifted to the right but it remains parallel (see Fig. 2.3).

Non-competitive antagonism

The effect of an agonist is reduced in the presence of the antagonist. No matter how much the dose of the agonist is increased it can not evoke a full response e.g. phenoxybenzamine and noradrenaline (see Fig. 2.4).

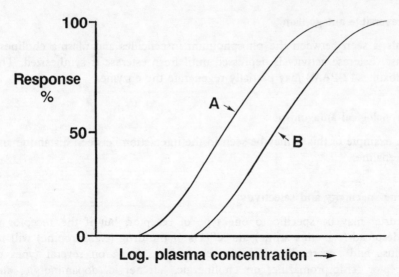

Fig. 2.3 Competitive antagonism. The dose–response curve of the agonist is shifted to the right (A to B), but a full response is still possible by increasing the dose of the agonist. A precise example is elusive, but curare (agonist) and neostigmine (antagonist) display this experimentally.

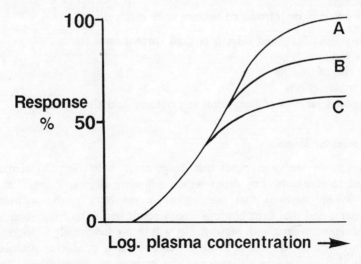

Fig. 2.4 Non-competitive antagonism. As the dose of antagonist is increased, the maximum response to the agonist falls from A to B to C.

Selective antagonism

Beta-adrenoreceptor blocking drugs may be non-selective, such as propranolol (blocks both $beta_1$ and $beta_2$). Atenolol is an example of a *selective antagonist*, blocking only $beta_1$ (the cardiac effects), reducing the risk of bronchoconstriction ($beta_2$). At high doses this selectivity may be lost.

Irreversible antagonism

This is seen between the phosphonium insecticides and plasma cholinest-erase. Esterase activity is depressed until fresh esterase is synthesized. The aldoximes (2-PAM) may partially regenerate the enzyme.

Physiological antagonism

An example of this is may be seen in the interaction between histamine and adrenaline.

Drug specificity and selectivity

A drug may be specific to one type of receptor, but if the receptor is widespread (e.g. muscarinic), the effects of the drug (e.g. atropine) will be diffuse and apparently non-selective. A drug acting on several types of receptor (chlorpromazine: on cholinergic, adrenergic, dopaminergic, and others) is non-specific. Atenolol is beta-specific and $beta_1$ selective.

New drugs

New drugs may be introduced because they display:

1. greater specificity and selectivity than current ones
2. new actions
3. less risk of toxicity
4. fewer side-effects
5. improved kinetics of absorption, distribution and elimination.

Drug–receptor kinetics

The occupation theory proposes that drugs exert their effects by remaining attached to receptors. For drugs which stimulate tissues, Paton (Paton & Payne 1968) proposed that stimulation occurs only at the moment of attachment, and that firm binding would result in the receptor then being blocked. Hence a drug with high affinity will be predominantly a blocker; one with lower affinity will attach, break free and re-attach, producing stimulation. This is the *rate theory*. It explains the actions of many drugs used in anaesthesia.

Acetylcholine (ACh) produces a rapid and intense action, limited to one millisecond by hydrolysis by cholinesterase. Inhibition of the esterase produces a cholinergic block, resistant to further doses of ACh. ACh has a high affinity, producing stimulation, and high attachment, producing block.

Suxamethonium is chemically similar to ACh, with high affinity and initial stimulation. Its slower hydrolysis reveals a high attachment, resulting in block. If this is prolonged, desensitization may result, in which the

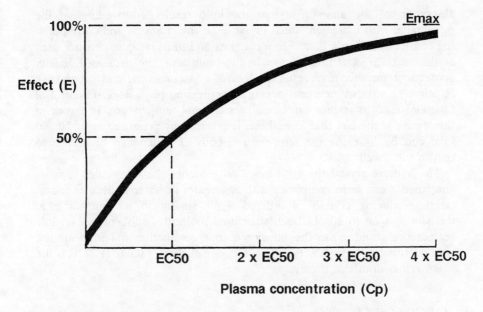

Fig. 2.5 Plasma concentration–effect. E_{max} is the maximum effect the drug can produce. EC_{50} is the concentration producing 50% of E_{max}. The graph is a hyperbola, but at plasma levels below EC_{50} the relationship is almost linear. There is a diminishing gain in effect for a given rise in concentration ($2 \times EC_{50}$, $3 \times EC_{50}$, $4 \times EC_{50}$); a reflection of the diminishing number of receptors available and an interesting demonstration of the law of mass action.

postjunctional membrane is insensitive to ACh. The intensity of this is dose-dependent, as is the time to recovery.

The **plasma concentration–effect relationship** (Fig. 2.5) is described by the **Michaelis–Menten expression:**

$$E = \frac{E_{max} \times Cp}{EC_{50} + Cp}$$

in which the effect (E) is related to the maximum effect (E_{max}), the actual plasma concentration (Cp) and the plasma concentration EC_{50} that produces 50% of the maximum effect (this is the affinity, see page 33). (Michaelis & Menten 1913).

THEORIES OF ANAESTHESIA

Overton and Meyer first related **lipid solubility** to effects of inhaled anaesthetics. The cell membrane is a lipid bi-layer enclosed between layers of protein, traversed by a number of globular proteins. The latter can aggregate to form micelles or channels usually comprising six molecules, through which ions pass when changes in excitability occur. It is thought that the absorption of the anaesthetic into the lipid results in 'swelling' of the membrane, with increased lateral pressure on the channels and corresponding restriction of ionic fluxes. In a complex and multisynaptic network such as the *reticular activating system* in the brainstem, the decreased activity consequent on this may result in loss of consciousness, and progressive impairment of other neuronal networks, depressing physiological control of functions such as respiration, blood pressure and temperature. In favour of this theory is the fact that anaesthesia is reversed by pressure (about 10 000 kPa) and by lowering the temperature, both of which can be shown to reduce the 'swelling'.

The **hydrate crystal theory** is based on evidence that molecules of some anaesthetics can form complexes with aggregates of water molecules (clathrates), producing crystals of ordered water similar to ice but stable at temperatures up to 30 °C. Such structured molecules adjacent to excitable membranes would impair the diffusion of ions, metabolites and other solutes, with depression of excitability. The absence of clathrates stable at 37°C is the major criticism of this theory.

MARGIN OF SAFETY

This is defined as:

$$\frac{\text{dose producing undesired or toxic effects}}{\text{dose producing therapeutic effects}}$$

A ratio of two or more is desirable so that susceptible patients will not become overdosed by dosage based on the need of the average patient.

Related to this is a ratio initially based on animal studies:

$$\text{Therapeutic index} = \frac{LD_{50}}{ED_{50}}$$

LD_{50} is the lethal dose which kills 50% of the animals, and ED_{50} is the effective dose which produces an effect in 50% of animals

UNEXPECTED OR UNPREDICTABLE EFFECTS

Idiosyncrasy is a genetically-determined extreme sensitivity or resistance to a drug, e.g. dibucaine-resistant plasma cholinesterase and duration of suxamethonium.

Hypersensitivity is an immune response to the drug (see Chapter 3).

Secondary effects are indirect consequences of the drug's action. Monoamine oxidase inhibitors inhibit the metabolism of amines in the gut wall. Ingested amines such as tyramine reach the circulation and act on sympathetic nerves to release noradrenaline, producing a hypertensive crisis.

TOLERANCE

The usual dose is ineffective and must be increased. Tolerance may be congenital or acquired. Racial and species tolerances are common, the latter limiting the usefulness of animal studies on drugs.

An interesting example of *acquired tolerance* is seen with *morphine*. Within 9 h of administration an increased metabolic degradation of the drug is seen. The commonest basis for acquired tolerance is *enzyme induction* in the liver, the *cytochrome P450* group of enzymes being involved. Related drugs may affect the metabolism of each other by the same mechanism, producing **cross-tolerance.**

The converse of this is the *inhibition of liver enzymes* by *cimetidine*, reducing drug metabolism and enhancing and prolonging the effects of many drugs e.g. warfarin.

Tachyphylaxis is a form of extreme tolerance. When an indirect sympath-omimetic drug (ephedrine) is given it releases noradrenaline. If noradrenaline is depleted by repeated large doses, a sharp fall in the response to the drug may occur.

COMBINED EFFECTS OF DRUGS

Synergism denotes an increase in the effect of a drug when another is given concomitantly (see Fig. 2.6). It may be *additive* when the total effect equals the sum of the individual effects: the two drugs usually act by a similar mechanism. *Potentiation* is said to occur when the combined response is greater than the sum of the individual responses: it may indicate varying modes of action e.g. tubocurarine blocks both pre-and postsynaptic cholin-ergic receptors, decreasing the amount of transmitter released and blocking it also. Alcuronium is a postsynaptic blocker only. A dose of tubocurarine

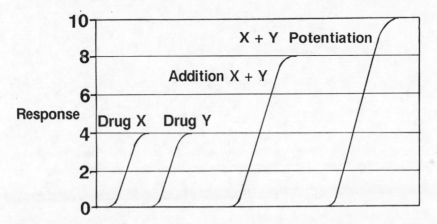

Fig. 2.6 Synergism. Addition: the combined effect of X and Y (8 units) is the sum of their individual effects (4 units). Potentiation: the response (10 units) is greater than the sum.

producing 25% block given with a dose of alcuronium producing 25% block results in measurably more than 50% block. Potentiation has also been applied to the enhancement of the effect of a drug by an unrelated drug e.g. chlorpromazine and morphine.

FURTHER READING

Michaelis M, Menten D L 1913 Die Kinetic der Invertinwirkung. Biochemische Zeitschrift 49: 333–369
Paton W D H, Payne J P 1968 Pharmacological Principles and practice. Churchill, London, p 3

3. Complications of drug therapy and interactions

Apart from the desired actions and known side-effects of drugs, there may be:

a. Unpredictable actions due to:
   1. hypersensitivity
   2. anaphylactoid responses
   3. genetic predisposition
b. Interactions with other drugs
c. Other complications.

UNPREDICTABLE ACTIONS

Hypersensitivity

This may occur only when a patient has received the drug before: an antigen–antibody reaction. Most drugs cannot act as antigens due to their low molecular weight, but complex with a protein to form a hapten, an active antigen.

Types of reactions

1. Anaphylaxis: The allergen acts on T and B lymphocytes, the latter producing plasma cells which synthesize and release IgE into the circulation. IgE has Fab and Fc portions. The Fc portion attaches to mast cells and basophils. On a second exposure to the allergen the Fab portions become cross-linked, altering the cell membrane and resulting in the release of intracellular autacoids (histamine, eosinophil chemotactic factors, heparin, kinins, 5-hydroxytryptamine (5-HT), slow-reacting substance A (SRS-A), prostaglandins E_2 and F_2-alpha, platelet-activating factor and lysosomal enzymes) (see Fig. 3.1). These cause smooth muscle contraction in the gut and bronchi, increased capillary permeability (oedema, urticaria) and relaxation in smaller blood vessels (hypotension, nasal obstruction and sneezing). The clinical onset is often marked by a violent cough.

Methiothepin is an antagonist to all three types of 5-HT_1 receptors. *Ketanserin* blocks 5-HT_2 receptors (in brain, uterus, aorta and platelets).

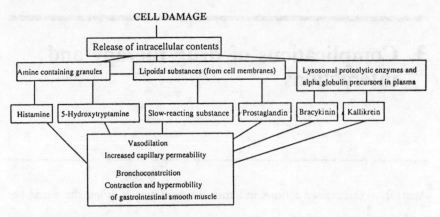

Fig. 3.1   Results of cell injury (secondary to anaphylaxis).

There are also specific antagonists to 5-HT$_3$ receptors in peripheral and autonomic nerves.

Mathieu and Kahan (1975) reported the following cases (number of cases in brackets): thiopentone (20), methohexitone (6), suxamethonium (6), d-tubocurarine (4). Fisher (1979) also reported alcuronium (7). (Other drugs which are now obsolete were also reported.) Other drugs commonly reported: penicillin, iodinated contrast media, dextran, foreign serum.

Anaphylaxis is treated with oxygen, i.v. adrenaline 1:10 000, pressor drugs, and hydrocortisone. Colloid solutions i.v. help sustain circulation in the face of increased capillary permeability: crystalloids are rapidly lost and may cause pulmonary oedema. Atropine reduces bronchial secretions and may reduce the severity of bronchoconstriction.

Tests for hypersensitivity (Fisher 1979) include:

a. Serum IgE level can be measured by a radio-absorbent test (RAST). A low value (<25 units/ml) suggests that allergy is unlikely; >100 units/ml indicates an allergic predisposition. A level >1 unit/ml in cord blood suggests that the newborn will be predisposed to allergy.

b. Intradermal skin test. 0.1 ml of 1:1000 dilution of the clinically-used solution. If negative, the strength of solution is increased and decreased tenfold and the test repeated. A positive test reveals histamine-releasing reactions, with wheal and flare. The test is delayed for a month after the reaction to enable autacoids to be replenished.

c. Basophil degranulation test. Mast cells incubated with immune serum become degranulated when exposed to the drug.

d. Prausnitz–Kustner test. The patient's serum is injected into a monkey. After 24 h the drug is injected at the same site. A flare and wheal indicate an immune response: an example of passive transfer of immunity by a 'reagin': IgE.

e. Lymphocyte transformation test. Lymphocytes from a sensitized animal divide when exposed to the drug.

f. Leucocyte migration inhibition. Sensitized leucocytes in culture become immobile when exposed to the drug.

2. Serum sickness-like reactions. Penicillin, sulphonamides.

3. Skin reactions. Phenothiazines may cause these but only with long exposure. Not reported with anaesthetic dosage.

4. Blood dyscrasias. Not reported with anaesthetics. A positive antinuclear factor may occur with alpha-methyl dopa.

Anaphylactoid responses

These may occur on *first exposure*, in contrast to anaphylaxis. They are less severe and shorter-lasting than anaphylaxis. Although not antigen–antibody reactions, they may be life-threatening due to hypotension and bronchospasm, together with erythema, urticaria, oedema and skin rashes.

Cremophor EL was used as a vehicle for drugs which are poorly water-soluble (propanidid, althesin) and was a common cause. It was the original vehicle for propofol but abandoned in favour of soya bean oil, egg phosphatide and glycerol as these are non-allergenic.

Complement activation is a feature of these responses: there are nine plasma proteins (C1–C9) which are activated sequentially (the classical complement pathway), releasing showers of biologically-active polypeptides (the anaphylatoxins). In turn these release vasoactive substances (mainly histamine) from mast cells and basophils.

Treatment

Discontinue the causative drug (if identified) and give oxygen. If oxygenation is normal, blood pressure does not fall and there is no history of previous exposure to the drug, no further measures may be necessary. If bronchospasm prevents ventilation, and blood pressure falls, treat as for anaphylaxis.

Note: A patchy or even generalized erythema is often seen after induction of anaesthesia. In children dTC very frequently causes a generalized flush, and atropine can cause red blotches. The likely cause is histamine release. The reaction is self-limiting and rarely outlasts the duration of the anaesthetic.

Genetic predisposition

Table 3.1 summarizes the more common 'pharmacogenetic' syndromes.

DRUG INTERACTIONS

Clinically significant interactions are uncommon in anaesthesia. They may be classified as:

Class I. Pharmaceutical: usually inactivation due to chemical or physical

Table 3.1 Genetic syndromes

Syndrome	Drug	Result	Genetic type	Incidence
Prolonged paralysis	Suxamethonium	Apnoea	Autosomal recessive	1:2800 (4% are heterozygous)
Malignant hyperthermia	Halothane Suxamethonium	Uncontrolled temperature rise	Autosomal dominant	1:20 000
Hepatic porphyria	Barbiturates	Abdominal pain Paralysis	Autosomal dominant	?
Slow or fast acetylators	Hydrallazine (no anaesthetics)	Slow: effects enhanced Fast: effects decreased	Autosomal recessive	40% of Caucasians are 'fast'
Glucose-6-phosphate dehydrogenase deficiency (Favism)	Aspirin Quinidine Sulphonamides Vitamin K	Haemolysis	Sex-linked dominant	108 in the world

incompatibility before reaching patient.

Class II. Pharmacokinetic: a drug alters the absorption, distribution, metabolism or excretion of another.

Class III. Pharmacodynamic: a drug enhances or depresses the actions of another by interacting at its site of action on or in the cell.

Class I: Pharmaceutical incompatibilities

These may be obvious: the precipitation of vecuronium by thiopentone (the precipitate redissolves in the blood and remains active). Less obvious is the adsorption of 40% of insulin to the walls of the container if it is added to i.v. fluids (this can be lessened by preliminary flushing with plasma protein solution). Adsorption to charcoal is a useful property when treating an overdose of paracetamol or a tricylic drug: it must be given within an hour of ingestion, before absorption is advanced.

With respect to additives to i.v. infusions: these questions should be asked:

1. Is it necessary to give the drug this way?
2. Is the drug stable when diluted with this fluid?
3. Are any other drugs added? Are they compatible?
4. Will the drug act in a highly diluted form?
5. Will the drug be adsorbed to the i.v. equipment and make the dosage unpredictable (see insulin above).

Class II: Pharmacokinetic interactions

Absorption from the gut is delayed by anticholinergic drugs (atropine), or enhanced by Maxolon which hastens gastric emptying. Maxolon may decrease the absorption of digoxin, which is slowly absorbed and undergoes too rapid a transit through the gut. Food usually delays drug absorption, but specific foodstuffs may have unexpected effects. Calcium in milk chelates tetracycline, slowing its absorption; paraffin oil is not absorbed and prevents the absorption of fat-soluble vitamins (A, D, E, K).

Gut mucosa contain *monoamine oxidase* which metabolizes amines during absorption. MAO inhibitors prevent this, allowing tyramine (from cheese, broad beans, beer) or phenylpropylamine (in cough mixtures) to reach the blood and produce an intense adrenergic effect (hypertensive crisis).

The *oral route* of administration has several disadvantages in anaesthesia:

1. slow absorption
2. uncertain rate of absorption
3. failure to absorb polar drugs
4. metabolism by first-pass before reaching the tissues.

Absorption from *subcutaneous injection* is slowed by addition of adrenaline to local anaesthetics, or by converting the drug to a less soluble form (procaine penicillin). An interesting pathophysiological kinetic interaction is seen in hypovolaemia following injury. Vasoconstriction delays the absorption of injected analgesic (morphine), and further doses may be given to attempt to achieve pain control. With resuscitation the circulation returns, with systemic absorption of the multiple doses and profound effects e.g. respiratory arrest. The problem is avoided by using the i.v. route.

Distribution from the blood is inhibited by plasma protein binding (PPB). Decreased plasma albumin increases the unbound fraction, and the greater availability to the tissues increases the effect of a dose. *Competition for PPB is important*: a patient stabilized on the anticoagulant warfarin may be prescribed phenylbutazone, this displaces some PPB warfarin leading effectively to overdose and haemorrhage (possibly intracranial). Conversely, withdrawing phenylbutazone may result in effective underdosage of warfarin, with the risk of thrombosis and embolism. Phenylbutazone can also displace the oral antidiabetic drug tolbutamide, leading to hypoglycaemia.

Drug metabolism is readily altered by additional drugs

1. *Phenobarbitone* causes enzyme induction of cytochrome P450 in hepatic microsomes, increasing the metabolism of many drugs. When given to a patient stabilized on warfarin, it results in lessened effectiveness of the warfarin. Conversely, when withdrawn the induction ceases and warfarin overdose may occur.

2. *MAO inhibitors* profoundly affect metabolism of drugs in the liver, brain, adrenergic neurones and other sites. The hypoglycaemic action of tolbutamide is increased. Pethidine may cause mania with hypertension or hypotension. Tricyclic antidepressants must be avoided as they inhibit the re-uptake of noradrenaline resulting in hyperpyrexia, twitching, flushing, hypertension

and unconsciousness. In general, the effects of drugs with amide groups are increased. MAO inhibitors have varied in usage. Some common ones are: tranylcypromine (Parnate), phenelzine (Nardil), iproniazid (Marsilid), isocarboxazid (Marplan).

3. *Plasma cholinesterase* hydrolyses esters (suxamethonium, procaine and, to some extent, atracurium). Cyclophosphamide or echothiopate (in eye drops) inhibit the enzyme and prolong the actions of the esters.

4. *Cimetidine* is a histamine$_2$ antagonist, but also inhibits drug metabolism in the liver. Warfarin, diazepam, phenytoin and propranolol are enhanced. It also reduces liver blood flow, reducing the extraction of many drugs (see Ch. 1, section 3).

Excretion

Probenecid competes with renal tubular transfer of acidic drugs. It lessens the reabsorption of uric acid, and the tubular excretion of penicillin: a clinically useful interaction.

Acidification of urine with *ammonium chloride* increases the excretion of pethidine and its metabolite, norpethidine.

Bleomycin, a cytotoxic drug, causes pulmonary fibrosis. The consequent restrictive defect slows the uptake and excretion of anaesthetic gases and vapours.

Class III. Pharmacodynamic interactions

a. Thiazide diuretics increase urinary potassium ion loss. Hypokalaemia increases the toxicity of digoxin, and the effect of non-depolarizing blockers.

b. Agonists and partial agonists are additive when given in small doses but partial agonists decrease the action of a full dose of agonist. Pentazocine (Fortral) is thus a partial agonist and weak antagonist (to morphine).

c. Aminoglycoside antibiotics (especially neomycin) increase non-depolarizing neuromuscular block by lessening ACh release; Mg^{2+} acts similarly. Hence Ca^{2+} reverses the block by about 70%; neostigmine reverses it by 20–67%. The action potential is prolonged by *4-aminopyridine* (Pymadin), increasing Ca^{2+} entry and ACh release, lessening the effect of the aminoglycoside. For the same reason 4-aminopyridine lessens the block in the Eaton–Lambert syndrome (seen in carcinoma of the lung).

d. Atropine and neostigmine are a familiar example of a useful pharmacodynamic interaction. Atropine blocks the unwanted muscarinic effects of the ACh, the duration of the latter being increased by the anticholinesterase.

e. Suxamethonium and non-depolarizing blockers. A small dose of a non-depolarizer (0.05 mg/kg of dTC) modifies the effects of suxamethonium in the following ways:

1. muscle fasciculations and pains are reduced
2. smaller rise in plasma K^+
3. smaller rise in intra-abdominal pressure.

These effects are useful in:

1. patients with a full stomach for urgent surgery (see note on dose below)
2. day-surgery cases, requiring early ambulation
3. patients with a history of severe muscle pains after suxamethonium.

Note: the *dose of suxamethonium must be increased to 1.5–2.0 mg/kg* to overcome the partial block. The intraocular pressure is raised following suxamethonium, an effect not modified by this technique (as was originally believed). For an open eye injury requiring emergency anaesthesia and intubation, it is now suggested that a large dose of a short-acting non-depolarizer (vecuronium 0.25 mg/kg or atracurium 1.25 mg/kg) is the safest means of achieving rapid paralysis.

f. Antihypertensive drugs are used very widely and are continued up to the time of anaesthesia to avoid rebound hypertension (especially seen with clonidine withdrawal). The decrease in vascular smooth muscle tone results in:

a. increased vasodilation during anaesthesia
b. poorer compensation for the effects of blood loss or changes of posture, e.g. head-up tilt.

With *beta-adrenoreceptor blockade bradycardia is also common,* with increased risk of episodes of hypotension.

g. Levodopa is widely used in the treatment of parkinsonism. It promotes the formation of dopamine in the CNS and peripherally. Bradycardia and ventricular dysrhythmias have been reported with halothane.

h. Inhaled anaesthetics and adrenaline. Halothane sensitizes the myocardium to catecholamines, limiting the use of adrenaline to 10 ml of 1:100 000 (given over 10 min) when combined local and general anaesthesia is used. Although the risk appears less with enflurane or isoflurane, caution should be used, and hypercapnea avoided as this causes a release of endogenous catecholamines.

OTHER COMPLICATIONS

Fever. Before ascribing a temperature rise to malignant hyperthermia, it is important to remember that fever may follow conventional dosage of: atropine, antiparkinsonian drugs (due to an anticholinergic effect), phenothiazines, some cytotoxic drugs, and surgical drapes which prevent evaporative heat loss (especially in small children). Less common causes are pyrogens in i.v. fluids and toxaemia from widespread infection.

Malignant hyperthermia is a particularly hazardous complication of inhalation anaesthesia. It may be genetically determined by an autosomal dominant gene (with a strong family history of anaesthetic deaths), or sporadic. *Halothane* has been most frequently implicated, but this complication has been reported with other inhalation agents. *Suxamethonium* is a common triggering agent. The syndrome is related to the changes in Ca^{2+} release and re-uptake by sarcoplasmic reticulum in muscle, the calcium channel responsible being the *ryanodine* receptor whose gene is located on the long arm of chromosome 19. There are probably other genetically related metabolic disorders which can cause the syndrome. *Dantrolene* is a specific antidote (1 mg/kg per minute, up to 10 mg/kg over 15 min). Its t½β is about 12 h. Prophylactic use is limited by side-effects of nausea and weakness in up to 70% of patients.

Purpura may be due to thrombocytopenia, platelet abnormalities, damage to blood vessels or anticoagulants. Anaesthetic-related drugs (atropine, lignocaine, dextran, diazepam, paracetamol) are fortunately rarely implicated.

Cytotoxic drugs are being increasingly encountered in anaesthetic practice. A list of the more important toxic effects follows:

1. *Adriamycin*: cardiac enlargement, low voltage ECG, cardiac output falls. Toxicity occurs at 500 mg/m^2.
2. *Arabinylcytosine*: respiratory insufficiency, hypoxaemia.
3. *Bleomycin*: painful muscles, pulmonary fibrosis (restrictive lung disease). Toxic dose is 250 mg/m^2.
4. *BCNU* (nitrogen mustard): pulmonary fibrosis.
5. *Cyclophosphamide*: pulmonary damage, lowered plasma cholinesterase.
6. *Hydroxyurea*: headache, convulsions.
7. *L-asparaginase*: liver damage, low fibrinogen and factor V, neurological disturbances.
8. *6-mercaptopurine*: liver damage, rarely pneumonitis.
9. *Methotrexate*: liver injury, somnolence, confusion, alveolitis.
10. *Mithramycin*: depresses liver and kidney function, may lower plasma Ca, P, K.
11. *Mitomycin C*: may depress liver and kidney function.
12. *Procarbazine*: weak MAO inhibitor, drowsiness or psychosis.
13. *Thiotepa*: depresses pseudocholinesterase.
14. *Vinblastine*: peripheral neuritis, headache, convulsions.
15. *Vincristine*: peripheral neuritis.

To minimize drug interactions:

1. A full history should be taken (see suggestions below).
2. Avoid multiple drug usage.
3. Take particular care with patients who are taking known interacting drugs: cimetidine, phenylbutazone, MAOIs, phenytoin.
4. Keep changes in drug therapy to a minimum, including stopping and restarting a drug.
5. Educate the patient in what is being taken and possible interactions.

A complete drug history should include:

1. proprietary (non-prescription) drugs
2. prescribed maintenance drugs
3. analgesics
4. vitamins
5. herbal and 'natural' remedies
6. Foodstuffs (e.g. tyramine in cheese) and additives:
   a. colouring agents
   b. preservatives (metabisulphite)
   c. flavouring
   d. antibacterials.

Fatal drug reactions

In a report (Shapiro et al 1971) of 744 fatalities of 6199 hospital admissions, drug reactions were contributory in 27:

5 from K$^+$ supplements (4 by infusion)
3 from opiates plus sedatives (chlorpromazine included)
3 from superinfection and septicaemia (with antibiotics)
2 from haemorrhage following heparin (of 361 cases)
1 from digitalis intoxication (of 1254 cases)
2 from diuretics: dehydration and electrolyte disturbance (of 1254 cases)
2 from hypoglycaemia (of 353 on insulin)
1 each from: neostigmine, adrenal steroids and 3 further drugs.

FURTHER READING

Fisher M McD 1979 Intradermal testing in the diagnosis of anaphylaxis during anaesthesia. Anaesthetics and Intensive Care 7: 58–61
Mathieu A Kahan B 1975 Immunological aspects of anaesthetic and surgical practice. Grune and Stratton, New York
Shapiro S, Slone D, Lewis G P, Jick H 1971 Fatal drug reactions among medical inpatients. Journal of the American Medical Association 216: 467

4. Premedication drugs except analgesics

DRYING AGENTS

Atropine was introduced in 1872 by Heidenhahn to suppress salivary and bronchial secretions especially during ether anaesthesia when these are profoundly stimulated. If it is used, there is no need to give it before induction when it can be given intravenously.

Scopolamine, in the dose of 8 µg/kg, is less effective as a vagolytic than atropine but has amnesic and sedative properties which have made it a useful premedicant. In this dose it suppresses salivation more than atropine 0.01 mg/kg, and patients may find this objectionable.

Glycopyrrolate is a synthetic drug with a shorter t½β. It suppresses secretions with minimal vagolysis.

Mechanism of action

The muscarinic effects of acetylcholine are antagonized non-competitively. They follow parasympathetic stimulation: vagal tone, salivary and bronchial secretions, decreased tone of sphincters, pupillary dilation. Cholinergic sympathetic nerves are also found: sweating and piloerection. The dose of atropine to block the vagus is less than that which suppresses salivation. At very high dosage atropine blocks autonomic ganglia and ultimately the neuromuscular junction (experimentally).

Sources and chemistry

Atropine is produced abundantly by the berries of *atropa belladonna* (deadly nightshade), and scopolamine by *hyoscyamus niger* (henbane). A number of other plants also produce both alkaloids. They are esters of tropic acid, with an organic base: tropine (atropine) or scopine (scopolamine). Atropine is a racemic mixture of d- and l-hyoscyamine (the d- form is inactive), and scopolamine is l-hyoscine. Both form water-soluble salts which arc very stable.

Glycopyrrolate is a synthetic quaternary amine and is highly polar. It is relatively expensive.

51

Administration

Subcutaneous or intramuscular injection of atropine takes 30 minutes to suppress secretions. *Intravenous (i.v.) injection* blocks the cardiac vagus in one circulation time, and secretions in 5–10 min.

Glycopyrrolate must be given by injection.

Oral: absorption of 90% of the dose occurs in the small bowel, but much of this is metabolized in the liver. With atropine eye-drops (1% or 10 mg/ml), enough to produce toxicity in small children may pass down the nasolacrimal ducts and then be swallowed.

Percutaneous absorption of scopolamine from the skin behind the ear has been used to control motion sickness. *Scop* is a transdermal therapeutic system containing 1.5 mg in a flat circular patch comprising 3 layers; 0.5 mg is released quickly from the adhesive, then 1.0 mg over 72 h from a membranous reservoir with controlled release. A skin-coloured, waterproof backing film seals the system.

Distribution

Atropine and scopolamine are widely distributed, including through the CNS. Glycopyrrolate, being polar, does not cross the blood–brain barrier.

Elimination

1. *Atropine*: plasma t½β 2.5 hours; 50% is excreted by the kidneys unchanged, but after i.v. injection, the proportion excreted unchanged rises from 50 to >70%; 85% is eliminated in 24 h.

2. Scopolamine is predominantly metabolized. Its maximum effect occurs during 1–2 h, but accommodation of vision may be affected for over 24 h.

3. Glycopyrrolate has a low distribution t½α (2–3 min) and elimination t½β (1–2 h) due to a low volume of distribution (0.66 l/kg) and high plasma clearance (0.5 l/kg per hour); 50% is excreted in 3 h and the drying effect lasts up to 8 h.

Actions

Toxicity. Atropine has a very wide margin of safety: recovery has occurred after 1000 times the normal dose in children. The main hazard is hyperthermia from suppression of sweating, but vasodilation predisposes to a loss of heat in a cold environment. Excitement and hallucinations occur: physostigmine antagonizes these effects as it also enters the CNS.

Cardiovascular system CVS. Tachycardia following atropine increases the cardiac output especially where this is rate-dependent (in children and in aortic stenosis) and may raise systolic and diastolic pressures slightly. The most significant effect is a shortening in the diastolic duration and a corresponding reduction of coronary blood flow and oxygen supply/demand ratio. This is particularly important in myocardial ischaemia. Peripheral venous tone falls and postural hypotension may occur. Atropine may cause ventricular dysrhythmias due to block of the AV node, especially during induction with halothane in children. Glycopyrrolate produces less tachycardia than atropine.

Respiratory system. Atropine dilates normal bronchi increasing physiological deadspace by 30%. Tidal volume increases to compensate. 0.012 mg/kg decreases flow resistance by 33% in normal bronchi. Scopolamine in clinical dosage is more effective as a drying agent.

CNS. Glycopyrrolate does not enter the CNS. Scopolamine is 5–15 times as potent as atropine: 0.4 mg causes amnesia in 35% of patients, and sedation is very common. Both atropine and scopolamine are weak antiemetics. Atropine-like drugs (Artane, Cogentin) are used in parkinsonism and the dystonic effects which may follow some phenothiazines and butyrophenones.

Gut. Atropine and scopolamine both lower the lower oesophageal sphincter tone, predisposing to oesophageal reflux. They reduce gastric acidity and pepsin secretion, but are less effective than histamine$_2$-receptor blockers (cimetidine, ranitidine, famotidine).

Eyes. Pupillary dilation (mydriasis) occurs and may persist for many hours, especially with topical use. Loss of accommodation (cycloplegia) follows paralysis of the ciliary body, with a similar duration.

Anticholinesterase poisoning. Large doses of atropine are necessary to block the excessive accumulation of ACh both in the CNS and peripherally. Aldoximes (2-PAM) may be partially successful in regenerating the cholinesterase, but up to 3 weeks are necessary for ACh to be restored. Anticholinesterases include malathion, dyflos, Sarin, Metasystox. They are used as pesticides and are readily absorbed by the skin, conjunctivae and lungs.

Final note. The use of premedicant drying drugs has decreased because:

1. irritant vapours are rarely used
2. their actions when given 1–2 h before anaesthesia are greatly decreased by the time anaesthesia is begun
3. when given i.v., tachycardia allows less myocardial perfusion
4. temperature regulation is impaired
5. patients dislike having a dry mouth
6. scopolamine may cause mania in elderly patients
7. scopolamine has been reported to cause intractable vomiting in up to 10% of children despite its normal antiemetic action
8. the tone of the lower oesophageal sphincter is reduced.

Their main roles in anaesthesia are therefore:

1. Controlling the bradycardia and salivation due to suxamethonium, particularly in repeated dosage.

2. Avoiding the reflex bradycardia which may follow traction on mesentery or vascular pedicles, or extraocular muscles.

3. Avoiding the bradycardia and salivation produced by neostigmine when reversing non-depolarizing neuromuscular block.

4. Providing sedation and amnesia (scopolamine), especially in major and prolonged procedures e.g. cardiac and faciomaxillary surgery.

5. Lessening the bradycardia which may occur with extensive regional analgesic techniques.

SLEEP AND SEDATIVES

Sleep

The *awake state* is maintained by the *reticular activating system, mid-brain and limbic system.* REM sleep comprises 25% of normal sleep: deprivation results in a feeling of tiredness (despite an adequate period of non-REM sleep), and is followed by an increase (rebound) of REM sleep. It is controlled by pontine nuclei whose transmitters are dopamine and noradrenaline. Fig. 4.1 shows the characteristic EEG patterns seen during sleep.

Daily sleep and the proportion of REM sleep vary during life.

The hours of sleep (REM proportion) are: 3 months, 14 h, (40%); 6 months, 13 h (30%); 3 years, 12h (25%); 6 years, 11 h (20%); 10 years, 10 h (18.5%); 15 years, 9 h (20%); 25 years, 8 h (22%); 35 years, 7 h (20%); 50 years, 6 h (20%); 90 years, 6 h (20%).

SEDATIVES

Sedatives are said to promote sleep, hypnotics to compel a desire for sleep: there is no distinct line between them. Both produce a feeling of tranquillity, and the term 'tranquillizer' has been applied to some members of this group of drugs (Oh & Duncan 1990).

Shortcomings of sedatives

1. May cause 'hangover' due to long t½β or active metabolites. Flurazepam has a brief t½β, being quickly converted to N-desalkylflurazepam, t½β, 47–100 h.

2. May suppress REM sleep.

3. When the sedative is stopped, rebound REM sleep occurs with increased dreams and feeling of unsatisfying sleep. Hence sedatives are resumed, and dependence results.

4. Become less effective with prolonged use.

5. Deliberate overdose may be used for suicide.

6. They may be misused to produce control of mild anxiety.

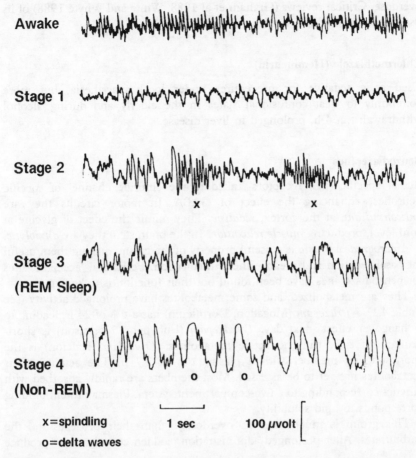

Awake

Stage 1

Stage 2

x   x

Stage 3
(REM Sleep)

Stage 4
(Non-REM)

o   o

x=spindling   1 sec   100 μvolt
o=delta waves

Fig. 4.1 EEG patterns during sleep. As sleep deepens, frequency falls and voltage increases. 'Spindles' are characteristics of REM sleep: 1 second bursts of 13–15 Hz. Delta waves appear in stage 3 and dominate stage 4.

Obsolete sedatives

These include barbiturates, due to dependence and suicide potential; methaqualone (Mandrax), due to euphoriant effect frequently leading to abuse and rapid onset of dependence.

Chloral hydrate

This has been widely used as a paediatric anaesthetic premedicant and a 'domiciliary' sedative. It does not suppress REM sleep or cause hangover; t½β 8 h. With chronic use dependence can develop. Disadvantages include an unpleasant taste, unpredictability of response and refractory arrhythmias in overdose. Critical reviews (Graham et al 1988, White and Whyte 1988) of its use in adults conclude that it is outmoded.

Chlormethiazole (Hemineurin)

Used as a sedative for procedures under local anaesthesia, but more commonly to treat confusional states in the elderly and during alcohol withdrawal; $t_{1/2}\beta$ 4 h, prolonged in liver disease.

Benzodiazepines

Act at specific (BZ) receptors linked to the chloride channel of specific neurones, enhancing the effect of GABA. In motor circuits they are *anticonvulsant*, at the cortex, *sedative*. They mimic the effect of glycine at cord level, producing *muscle relaxation*. In the brain stem they are *anxiolytic*.

Anterograde amnesia is a useful property of the group, making them useful for basal sedation and preanaesthetic medication. Peripheral 'acceptor' sites for benzodiazepines have been found but their function is unknown.

They are metabolized, and some metabolites have prolonged activity (see Table 4.1). *Nitrazepam* (Mogadon, Dormicum) has a $t_{1/2}\beta$ of 24 h, leading to a 'hangover effect' next day. *Temazepam* (Euhypnos, Normison) is short-acting, $t_{1/2}\beta$ 8 h, with no active metabolites. *Triazolam* (Halcion) is the shortest-acting member with a plasma $t_{1/2}\beta$ of 2.7 h. The activity of its metabolites has yet to be assessed. Most members are rapidly absorbed with kinetics corresponding to a two-compartment system. Plasma protein binding corresponds to lipid solubility.

This group is much safer in overdosage than their predecessors, the barbiturates. After prolonged administration, sudden cessation may produce

Table 4.1 Benzodiazepines: half-lives and metabolism

Drug	Data	$t_{1/2}\beta$, hours	Metabolism
Diazepam (Valium)	Volume of distribution (Vd) 0.7–1.7 l/kg Plasma protein binding (PPB) 99%	24–50 90 at 80 years	Hepatic metabolism to oxazepam and desmethyl-diazepam: $t_{1/2}\beta$ 50–120 h
Oxazepam (Serepax)	PPB 96%	6–8	Hepatic metabolism to inactive glucuronide
Temazepam (Euhypnos)		6–8	Inactive metabolites
Nitrazepam (Mogadon, Dormicum)		18–34	Genetic variability in further metabolism of amine metabolite
Midazolam (Hypnovel)	Vd 1.1–1.7 l/kg PPB 97%	1.7–4	Hepatic metabolism to hydroxymethyl-midazolam may prolong action
Lorazepam	PPB 90%	9–16	Hepatic metabolism to inactive glucuronide

withdrawal effects: depression, agitation, tremor, cramps, insomnia and vomiting. Some degree of tolerance may develop, and cross-tolerance to other sedatives may occur: e.g. alcohol, chloral. When taken together, alcohol and the benzodiazepines may produce an enhanced effect: errors in motor driving or other skilled tasks may occur.

Midazolam is the only water-soluble member and hence the most suitable for i.v. use. When given i.v., it may depress the CO_2 response. This may result in apnoea, especially in the elderly. Care must be taken to monitor the patient. Its slow onset of action predisposes to overdosage: it must be given in small increments, with pauses for the effects to develop.

Note. i. Oral midazolam in dosage 0.5–0.75 mg/kg has been recommended for day-surgery premedication in children.

ii. Induction of anaesthesia with midazolam is 'unsuccessful' in 14% of patients because:

a. the range of dosage is very wide

b. onset is slow: 5–10 min

c. onset of unconsciousness is difficult to identify: the eyes may be open and the patient responding to command but there may be no memory of this.

Midazolam is reviewed by Reves et al (1985).

Flumazenil (Anexate)

This is an imidazodiazepine which is a specific benzodiazepine receptor antagonist. Its t½β is 60 min, clearly much shorter than any of the benzodiazepines. It may need to be given in repeated dosage or infusion if reversal is to be maintained. Its relative kinetics thus resemble those of naloxone whose t½β is also about 60 min, shorter than those of morphine or pethidine. It is expensive.

Buspirone

This is a recently introduced new class of anxiolytic which appears to be free of dependency and withdrawal problems. Its slow onset makes it unsuitable for use in anaesthetics.

Tranquillizers

Many sedative drugs are called tranquillizers because they also allay anxiety. Anxiety is one of the beta-effects of adrenaline, with symptoms such as palpitations, tremor and gastrointestinal upset which can be reduced by small doses of beta-adrenoreceptor antagonists e.g. propranolol. This has been used by performers, e.g. musicians, and in anaesthetic premedication. It also enhances the induction of deliberate hypotension.

ANTIEMETICS

The *vomiting centre* in the medulla has ACh and histamine$_1$-receptors. The *chemoreceptor trigger zone* in the area postrema (floor of the 4th ventricle) has dopamine$_2$-receptors. Table 4.2 shows the afferent neural inputs into the vomiting centre and the site of action of the antiemetic drugs.

Metoclopramide and domperidone lessen vomiting by increasing the rate of gastric emptying and increasing the tone of the lower oesophageal sphincter. Metoclopramide is a benzamide and is given orally or by injection. Its t½β is 2.5–5 h; 80% is excreted to the urine in 24 h, 50% being conjugated; plasma protein binding (PPB) 15%. It is a dopamine receptor antagonist and also causes a rise in prolactin and aldosterone, and mild sedation. The incidence of extrapyramidal effects is 1%, but these are more common in children, and may follow a single dose.

The 5-hydroxytryptamine-3 (5-HT-3) antagonist *ondansetron* (Zofran) appears to be more specific and avoids extrapyramidal side-effects. It is thought to inhibit the effects of 5-HT on the gut and the area postrema and is being used during cytotoxic treatment. After i.v. injection its t½β is 2.5–6 h.

Phenothiazines: chlorpromazine (Largactil) has a mild antiemetic action, but the piperazine-substituted phenothiazine *prochlorperazine* is more effective. It has a long t½β, possibly due to enterohepatic recirculation. It is a weak antagonist of alpha-adrenoreceptors, ACh, histamine and hydroxytryptamine, leading to hypotension, sedation and impaired temperature control. It also causes extrapyramidal reactions. Thiethylperazine (Torecan) is reported to have fewer side-effects than prochlorperazine.

Butyrophenones: droperidol causes dysphoria, sedation, hypotension and occasionally extrapyramidal movements. A low dose (e.g. 1.25 mg) still effectively inhibits vomiting and minimizes these side-effects. This is given i.v. during anesthesia. It is long-acting, with t½β 130 min. It is excreted in both urine and bile, 50% being unchanged.

Table 4.2   Vomiting: input and control

	Afferents	Source	Drugs

Vomiting centre	Higher centres
	8th cranial nerve
	  (vestibular)
	Vagus nerve
	Spinal cord via
	  sympathetics
	Chemoreceptor
	  trigger zone
		Pain, emotion
		Movement
		Gut, biliary tree, heart,
		  lungs
		Stomach, peritoneum,
		  genitourinary tract
			Scopolamine, some
			  antihistamines

Chemoreceptor
  trigger zone
	No neural input	Radiation sickness
		Opiates
		Anaesthetics
		Ergometrine
		Digoxin
		Tumour chemotherapy
			Phenothiazines, some
			  antihistamines,
			  butyrophenones,
			  metoclopramide,
			  domperidone,
			  ondansetron

Antihistamines: promethazine (Phenergan – also a phenothiazine) is a long-acting agent which also has sedative and anticholinergic actions. These properties also make it useful as a premedicant. *Cyclizine* also has anticholinergic actions but has minimal side-effects.

Anticholinergics: scopolamine, and *atropine* to a lesser extent, depress the vomiting centre, but the effect is much less than the agents mentioned above.

ANTACIDS

Alkalis will neutralize gastric acid if adequate mixing occurs. However, sodium bicarbonate when reducing acidity produces sodium chloride that then enhances acid production. *Sodium citrate* is preferable (30 ml of 0.3 molar solution). It is given less than an hour before anaesthesia as its duration of action is short. *Magnesium trisilicate* produces a floccular precipitate with acid which can cause a chemical pneumonitis, and it is used decreasingly.

Histamine$_2$ antagonists suppress gastric acid production. Injection i.v. raises pH to >2.5 in 30 min, orally it takes 3 h. *Cimetidine* (Tagamet) reduces hepatic blood-flow (a possible risk factor with halothane), and it also antagonises cytochrome P450 enzymes in the liver, enhancing the effects of warfarin, propranolol and phenytoin. *Ranitidine* (Zantac) and *famotidine* (Pepcidine) are reported to be free of this interaction.

OTHER DRUGS

Clonidine (Catapres) is a central alpha$_2$-adrenoreceptor stimulant which decreases the hypertensive response to tracheal stimulation, lowers anaesthetic MAC and is also reported to lessen anxiety preoperatively. Its t½β exceeds 12 h. It can be given orally. Its hypotensive action may be a hazard to patients with cerebrovascular disease. It has also been given transdermally.

FURTHER READING

Graham S R, Day R O, Lee R, Fulde G W O 1988 Overdose with chloral hydrate. Medical Journal of Australia 149: 686–688
Oh T E, Duncan A W 1990 Sedation in the seriously ill. Medical Journal of Australia 152: 540–545
Reves J G, Fragen R J, Vinik H R, Greenblatt D J 1985 Midazolam: pharmacology and uses Anesthesiology 62: 319–324
White A J, Whyte I M 1988 New Drugs for old. Medical Journal of Australia 149: 581–582

5. Analgesics

HISTORY

Opium dates from 3500 BC. Its preparations were crude until Serturner isolated morphine in 1803, Robiquet codeine and Pelletier papaverine and other alkaloids in 1832. Addiction became common when hypodermic injection became widely available in the 1880s. Heroin was made by Wright in 1884: addiction rapidly followed, but synthesis of heroin marked the start of a search for an analgesic drug free from central depression and addiction.

OPIOIDS

All naturally-occurring and synthetic drugs with *morphine-like* actions are known as *opioids*. Morphine, with its long history, is central in our knowledge of these drugs and is the standard for comparison. Now that opiate receptors have been defined, a more modern definition is that *any drug that binds to an opiate receptor as an agonist is classified as an opioid*. Opioids may be classified according to their action on the opiate receptor or according to their method of production or source (see Tables 5.1 and 5.2).

Mechanism of action: the opiate receptors

Three opiate receptors have been defined in man, related to the following effects:

- **mu:** supraspinal analgesia, euphoria, respiratory depression, meiosis, physical dependence, prolactin release
- **kappa:** spinal analgesia, respiratory depression, sedation, meiosis
- **sigma:** dysphoria, hallucinations, vasomotor stimulation.

Note: Further research into receptor subtypes with the goal of producing a drug with selective analgesia without respiratory depression has not been fruitful. Opioid peptides and exogenous opioids have different receptor affinities just as adrenergic agonists adrenaline, noradrenaline and isoprenaline have different affinities for alpha- and beta-adrenoreceptors. Two other opiate receptors, *delta* (endogenous agonist: leu-enkephalin) and *epsilon*

Table 5.1 Classification of opioids: Action on opiate receptor

Agonists	Antagonists	Agonist/antagonists
Morphine	Naloxone	Nalorphine
Pethidine	Naltrexone	Pentazocine
Fentanyl		Butorphine
Alfentanil		Nalbuphine
Sufentanil		Buprenorphine

Table 5.2 Classification based on method of production or source

Naturally occurring (Papaver somniferum)	Semisynthetic	Synthetic	Endogenous
Morphine	Heroin (diacetylmorphine)	Phenylperidine	Pro-opiomelanocortin (α, β and γ-endorphins)
Codeine (methylmorphine)	Dihydromorphinone	pethidine	Prodynorphin
Thebaine	Thebaine derivatives	fentanyl	Proenkephalin
Papaverine		alfentanil	(met- and leu-enkephalin)
		sufentanil	
		ketocyclazine	
		Methadone	
		Pentazocine	
		Levorphanol	

(agonist: beta-endorphin), have been identified in animals, but evidence for their existence in man is lacking.

Opioids also vary in their *efficacy* (the fraction of receptors occupied to produce an effect). High efficacy: sufentanil, fentanyl; low efficacy: morphine, pethidine. Opiate antagonists also show *selectivity* for different receptors (see Table 5.3).

Table 5.3 Opiate receptors

Antagonist	mu	kappa	sigma
Naloxone	Antagonist	Antagonist	Antagonist
Nalorphine	Antagonist	Partial agonist	Agonist
Naltrexone	Antagonist		
Partial agonist: Agonist/antagonist equivalent dose in mg			
Buprenorphine (0.3)	Partial agonist		
Dezocine (10)	Partial agonist		
Nalbuphine (10)	Partial agonist	Agonist	Agonist
Pentazocine (40)	Partial agonist	Agonist	Agonist
Agonist (equivalent dose in mg)			
Morphine (10)	Agonist	Agonist	
Butorphanol (2)	Agonist	Agonist	

STRUCTURE–ACTIVITY RELATIONSHIPS

Features common to opioids (see e.g. Fig. 5.1 morphine):

1. phenolic group, attached to
2. quaternary carbon (13), followed by
3. two carbon atoms (15, 16) and
4. amine group (17).

Substitutions

1. 3-OH, 17-N-CH$_3$: morphine (see Fig. 5.1).
2. 3-CH$_3$: decreased analgesia and respiratory depression; increased central stimulation. Example: codeine.
3. 3,6-OCH$_3$: increased central stimulation and excitation. Example: heroin (diacetylmorphine).
4. 17-N-allyl: partial agonist (agonist/antagonist). Example: nalorphine.
5. 6 = O, 3-OH: oxymorphones. Examples: naloxone (17-CH$_2$CH = CH$_2$), naltrexone.
6. Absence of 4,5 ether: morphinans. Example butorphanol.
7. Absence of 4,5 ether: absence of C6,7: benzomorphans. Example: pentazocine.

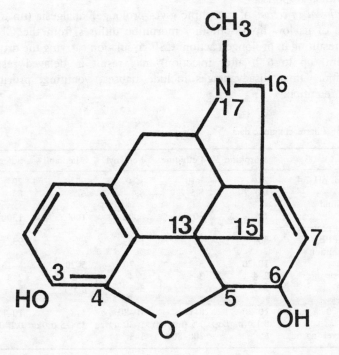

Fig. 5.1 Morphine.

8. Basic structure only: phenylpiperidines. Examples: pethidine, fentanyl, alfentanil, sufentanil.

Note:

1. Phenanthrenes have 5 rings, (as in morphine), morphinans 4, benzomorphans 3 and phenylpiperidines 2 rings.
2. Replacing the 17N-methyl with an allyl group results in an antagonist: morphine/nalorphine, oxymorphone/naloxone, levorphanol/levallorphan.

MORPHINE

Pharmacokinetics (See Table 5.4)

Oral bioavailability is only 15–30% due to its high ionization (80% at pH 7.4), low lipid solubility and first-pass metabolism. It can be given sublingually but has an unacceptable taste.

Bolus 0.1–0.2 mg/kg + infusion 10–30 µg/kg per hour is used to avoid peaks and troughs (respiratory depression or inadequate analgesia) which may result from 4-hourly doses (see Figs 1.1.1 and 1.1.2). *Patient-controlled analgesia (PCA)* with limited doses available on demand at regulated intervals is used to this effect. Careful monitoring is essential because of the variation in individual response.

Intrathecal injection of morphine gives prolonged analgesia (up to 24 h). Because of its low lipid solubility morphine diffuses from the CNS very slowly, resulting in prolonged action. CSF circulation carrying the drug to the brainstem (up to 6 h after injection) may result in delayed respiratory depression. Other disadvantages include nausea, vomiting, pruritus and urinary retention.

Table 5.4   Pharmacokinetic data

	Morphine	Pethidine	Fentanyl	Alfentanil	Sufentanil
% Ionized, pH 7.4	23	<10	<10	90	20
pKa	8.0	8.5	8.4	6.5	8.0
Relative lipid solubility	1	30	600	100	1300
% Plasma protein binding (PPB)	30	70	84	92	93
$t_{1/2}\alpha$ distribution (minutes)	10–20	5–15	5–20	5–20	5–15
$t_{1/2}\beta$ (hours)	2–4	3–5	2–4	1–2	2–3
Vd (1/kg)	3–5	3–5	3–5	0.5–1	2.5
Clearance (ml/min, 70 kg patient)	10–20	8–18	10–20	3–8	10–12
Dose i.v.	0.15 (mg/kg)	1.5 (mg/kg)	1–30 µg/kg	25–75 µg/kg	0.1–0.2 µg/kg
Plasma level (ng/ml)	65	200–800	1–3		

pKa is the pH at which 50% of the drug is ionized

Epidural injection results in transfer of morphine to the subarachnoid space and a prolonged effect. After a 10 mg injection, maximum ventilatory depression may occur after 10 h and still be detectable after 22 h. With other more lipid-soluble drugs, systemic uptake is quicker, resulting in a shorter duration of action. If longer duration of action is desired (e.g. postoperative analgesia) administration by infusion is more suitable than bolus.

Distribution

Only 0.1% enters the CNS after i.v. injection despite the low PPB (30%, compared with alfentanil 92%). It distributes in all tissues. It is then concentrated in the liver on the endoplasmic reticulum. Here it is demethyl-ated to normorphine, the 6-glucuronide (which is active) and the 3-glucuronide (inactive). The kidneys excrete 60–90% as morphine, normor-phine and the glucuronide conjugates. About 5% is metabolized to CO_2.

Pharmacodynamics

CNS: Stimulant effects produce nausea, vomiting (chemoreceptor trigger zone), meiosis (3rd cranial nerve nucleus) and may cause mania. A fall in blood pressure results from depression of vasomotor centre. This is enhanced by vasodilation from histamine release, and some adrenoreceptor blocking activity. Reflex circulatory responses to changes of posture are impaired. The respiratory centre is depressed, the respiratory rate slowed, the CO_2 response curve shifts to the right (i.e. less response to rises in inspired CO_2). Arterial CO_2 rises. Sympathetic discharge may cause hyperglycaemia. Cholinesterase is partly inhibited.

Gut: increased tone in sphincters and bowel wall; reduced peristalsis and constipation results. No tolerance develops to these effects (nor to meiosis).

Lungs: depresses cough, produces bronchoconstriction and reduces ciliary activity.

Antidiuretic hormone release increases.

Dependence and tolerance: occur quickly, but less so in patients who have pain. Abstinence or naloxone precipitate withdrawal effects (agitation, abdominal cramps, lacrimation). This is a hazard when dependence is unsuspected and also in babies of dependent mothers. Morphine dependence can continue for years, the individuals being quiet, withdrawn and passive but socially competent. A greater hazard of dependence and deterioration of personality appears to accompany heroin use.

PAPAVERETUM (Omnopon)

A mixture of opium alkaloids: 50% morphine (80% of activity). The contribution of shorter half-life alkaloids results in a t½ of about 3.5 h compared with morphine (about 4 h).

CODEINE

Methylmorphine. Bioavailability is 50%, and 20% is converted to morphine in the liver and can lead to dependence. Mostly excreted unchanged by the kidney. Its dosage is limited (8–30 mg) in non-prescription analgesics such as panadeine (paracetamol 500 mg, codeine 8 mg).

PETHIDINE (Meperidine, Demerol)

A piperidine derivative whose analgesic properties were discovered by chance in 1939 when anticholinergic drugs were being developed.

Pharmacokinetics (See Table 5.4)

Oral bioavailability is 56%, but rises to 90% in cirrhosis. Clearance falls by 25% postoperatively and by 50% in cirrhosis, and cimetidine reduces it by reducing liver blood flow and metabolism. Phenytoin induces liver enzymes, increasing clearance by 25%.

4% is excreted in urine unchanged or as norpethidine. If urine is acidified (2 g ammonium chloride 6-hourly), 22% is excreted unchanged and 24% as norpethidine, reducing its $t\frac{1}{2}\beta$. In the presence of monoamine oxidase inhibitors (tranylcypromine, iproniazid) its metabolism is impaired, and the patient may become confused, excited or depressed, and hypotension may occur. These effects are probably related to an accumulation of norpethidine, a proconvulsant. Excitement may be controlled with chlorpromazine and corticosteroids. Norpethidine is also formed in the CSF with epidural or subarachnoid injection of pethidine, and toxic levels have been reported. CSF $t\frac{1}{2}\beta$ for pethidine is 70 min.

FENTANYL (Sublimaze)

Pharmacokinetics (See Table 5.4)

Its high fat solubility results in rapid entry to the CNS and short duration of action due to redistribution. A second peak in the plasma concentration appears to be related to its accumulation in the acidic cells of the stomach (it is a basic amine) and in lipid stores, with subsequent release. This becomes significant if large doses have been given as delayed respiratory depression may result. It diffuses rapidly through the dura when given by epidural injection but is also taken up by extradural fat.

It is metabolized to norfentanyl (inactive) and further hydroxylated and excreted by the kidney.

Pharmacodynamics

As well as its profound analgesic effects, in higher dosage (30 µg/kg) it can produce anaesthesia, and this action combined with minimal effects on the cardiovascular system has led to its use in cardiac anaesthesia.

ALFENTANIL (Alfenta)

Pharmacokinetics (See Table 5.4)

The lower Vd and pKa increase the rate of onset and shorten its duration of action, making it more suitable as an opioid anaesthetic. Caution must be taken in patients who take alcohol regularly as they may require up to twice the dosage.

METHADONE

A synthetic drug which lasts 6–8 h and has 80% bioavailability. Its long life can lead to overdose and limits its use in anaesthesia. It is used to treat narcotic dependence.

PENTAZOCINE (Fortral)

A partial agonist (derived from phenazocine, which causes dysphoria). In its racemic form (d+,l–), 30 mg are equivalent to 10 mg morphine. Up to 87% is metabolized, but variations affect the predictability of analgesia. Side-effects include euphoria, dependence, sweating and tachycardia. It can be given orally. The cardiovascular effects in patients with coronary artery disease are important: after i.v. injection rises occur in plasma adrenaline, mean aortic pressure, left ventricular end-diastolic pressure, pulmonary artery pressure and the work of the heart.

BUPRENORPHINE (Temgesic)

A longer-acting partial agonist which is absorbed sublingually with 55% bioavailability. Analgesia persists despite a decline in plasma level, indicating slow association and dissociation constants, in keeping with the rate theory of drug action on receptors.

OXYCODONE

A semisynthetic opiate which is used increasingly in the treatment of terminal pain in cancer. Proladone is the pectinate and is well absorbed from suppositories, lasting about 8 h. Endone is the hydrochloride and may be given orally 6-hourly.

ENDOGENOUS OPIOIDS

Enkephalins and endorphins are polypeptide fragments of beta-lipotropin, a peptide from the anterior pituitary gland with a precursor which is common to ACTH.

Note: They are derived from the last 31 amino acids as follows: 61–76 (alpha-endorphin), 61–91 (beta-endorphin), 61–77 (gamma-endorphin) and 61–65 (met-enkephalin). Dynorphin is leucine-enkephalin. Opiate receptors and the opioids are found in the substantia gelatinosa of the cord, the tractus solitarius (related to respiratory and circulatory effects of opiates), periaqueductal grey matter, medial thalamic nuclei, amygdala, posterior pituitary, and in peripheral tissues such as the myenteric plexus and endocrine organs.

To obtain effective analgesia with minimal side-effects, vigorous research efforts are being directed to the production of analgesics which are opiate-receptor specific, and drugs, e.g. kelatorphin, which inhibit the breakdown of endogenous opioids which otherwise are rapidly metabolized.

COMPARISON OF ANALGESICS

When comparing analgesic drugs the following points are important:

1. Pain due to injury is preferable to experimentally-induced pain.
2. Bias should be avoided by 'blindness'.
3. A dose–response curve should be found for each drug.
4. Proper statistical analysis of results is essential.
5. Side-effects are best assessed in healthy volunteers.
6. Studies require full-time attention and do not mix easily with clinical responsibility.
7. Adequate controls are important: morphine as an effective agent and saline as a placebo.
8. Analgesia should not be confused with sleep.
9. Side-effects should be measured with equianalgesic doses.
10. Safety of patients and volunteers is essential.

Tests for pain

1. Radiation of a skin area with a laser. This stimulates a number of pain fibres and reveals effects on spinal and central processing of pain such as summation, facilitation and occlusion.
2. Pressure on the subcutaneous surface of the tibia.
3. Electrical stimulation of tooth pulp.
4. Ischaemic pain following application of a tourniquet.

Measurement of pain

Linear pain score. The patient is asked to grade the severity on a scale of 1–10 from no pain to unbearable pain. More consistent results have been obtained than when the severity is verbally described (slight, moderate, severe).

Note: pain has an emotional content, which explains why both analgesics and placebos are more effective in clinical than experimental pain. Chlorpromazine lessens the emotional effect, making it a useful adjunct in clinical practice.

THERAPEUTIC USES OF ANALGESICS

Opioid analgesics raise the threshold to pain, in contrast to antipyretic-type analgesics. Increasing knowledge of pain receptors and related agonists and antagonists have broadened this area of pharmacology, making current reviews the best source of information.

Intramuscular injection. The unpleasantness of injection and short half-lives of most analgesics has led to a preference for alternative methods of administration.

Drug infusions may be given into an i.v. drip or subcutaneously using the kinetics of absorption and elimination to obtain a plasma level within the effective range and avoiding peaks and troughs. It is necessary to give a loading dose to produce an effective level (see section 1.1).

Epidural injection of opioids is widely used. The drugs penetrate the dura at a rate proportional to their lipid solubility: pethidine and fentanyl faster than morphine. For the same reason their duration of action is briefer as they diffuse out of the dura equally readily. They may be added to local anaesthetics to enhance the duration and quality of analgesia.

Subarachnoid injection of opioids enables small doses of drugs to provide profound analgesia of long duration with fewer side-effects than result from parenteral use. Caution must be taken as the circulation of CSF is slow, and the effects of the opioid on the brain stem (respiratory depression especially) may be delayed for hours but may be profound.

Sublingual absorption. This route avoids first-pass metabolism and is effective for buprenorphine and nalbuphine. Morphine is also well absorbed, but its unpleasant taste makes it unacceptable.

Oral administration is unreliable with most agents due to variable absorption and first-pass metabolism. Methadone is effective and has a long duration of action, but efforts to adapt it for anaesthetic practice have not been successful.

Note: Old age. Susceptibility to morphine increases, and dosage may be reduced by 30% at 70 years and 50% at 80 years.

SIDE-EFFECTS

Respiratory depression is the most hazardous. The CO_2-response curve is shifted to the right, reflecting the lowered sensitivity of the respiratory centre to CO_2. Respiratory rate falls and respiratory acidosis develops.

Vomiting is a common and distressing problem. Antiemetics are of limited effect in controlling it. It is commoner when opioid analgesics are used in surgery on the eye muscles and some other sites, leading to the preferred use of antipyretic analgesics, or administration of the opioids to restricted sites e.g. epidural injection.

Meiosis occurs due to 3rd cranial nerve stimulation. Although tolerance to some of the actions of morphine develops, meiosis and constipation continue.

Sleep disturbance occurs in pain-free volunteers with suppression of REM sleep. It is believed that this contributes to the tiredness often seen during the first few days after surgery.

Pruritus: 1% after systemic morphine, 10% with epidural and 45% with subarachnoid injection. Not related only to histamine release (which produces itchiness of the nose with systemic injection).

NON-STEROIDAL ANTI-INFLAMMATORY DRUGS (NSAIDS, see Table 5.5)

Inflammatory mechanisms

Prostaglandins are synthesized by most cells and act locally as **tissue hormones.** They are derived from arachidonic acid, especially under the stimulus of vasoactive peptides (angiotensins, kinins). They may be tissue-specific: prostacyclin (PGI_2) dilating blood vessels, thromboxane (TXA_2) aggregating platelets, PGE_2 transporting epithelia in the alimentary and urinary tracts. They mediate inflammation and arthritis, inhibit gastric acid secretion and increase mucus production, and enhance the repair of alimentary injury by increasing the migration of cells. NSAIDS thus have a complex effect on the responses to surgery.

Pharmacokinetics

Administration is by mouth or rectally, limiting their usefulness postoperatively until the recent introduction of i.v. ketorolac and lysine acetylate (LAS). They are unpalatable, especially paracetamol. Aspirin is trapped in gastric

Table 5.5 Non-steroidal anti-inflammatory drugs NSAIDS *Note:* All NSAIDS are highly plasma protein-bound. **Paracetamol** is not strictly an NSAID as it is not anti-inflammatory, and it is less protein-bound.

Drug	Dose (mg/kg)	pKa	Duration (hours)	Metabolism
Acetylsalicylic acid (Aspirin)	15.00	3.5	6	To glucuronide, also excreted as free acid, enhanced by urine pH >7.5
Paracetamol (Panadol)	10.00	9.5	4	To glucuronide and sulphate
Indomethacin (Indocid)	0.50		8	Partly to glucuronide: complex excretion
Diclofenac (Voltaren)	0.50		8	50% first-pass: hydroxylation and to glucuronide
Piroxicam (Feldene)	0.15		24	95%, by hydroxylation and to glucuronide
Naproxen (Naprosyn)	7.00		6	40% to glucuronide, 30% demethylated

mucosa, causing local injury and bleeding. The other agents are less prone to cause this, but side-effects are common and limit their usefulness.

Pharmacodynamics

These drugs are used increasingly to control pain, often as adjuvants to the opiates (Dahl & Kehlet 1991). They act by preventing the synthesis of prostaglandins from arachidonic acid. **Salicylates** permanently acetylate cyclo-oxygenase, preventing prostaglandin endoperoxide synthesis: the inhibition by other NSAIDS is reversible (Weismann 1991). **Paracetamol** blocks prostaglandin synthetase in the CNS only and is antipyretic but not anti-inflammatory (it is not a true NSAID). Some other NSAIDS e.g. indomethacin inhibit phosphodiesterase, increasing the intracellular cyclic AMP and stabilizing cell membranes, and decreasing the release of kinins. For *optimal effects* the NSAIDS should be *given prior to the onset of pain*.

Side-effects

These arise mainly from the inhibition of cyclo-oxygenase but toxic ones are important also. **Prolonged bleeding time** due to reduced platelet adhesion and aggregation after aspirin is a hazard especially in ENT surgery in children. **Gastric ulceration**, gastritis and **depression of renal function** have limited the wider use of the group perioperatively.

Overdose: paracetamol causes **liver injury** by producing a reactive intermediate alkylating metabolite which exceeds the capacity of glutathione to inactivate it. Aspirin produces a **metabolic acidosis** and has been associated with **asthma**.

FURTHER READING

Dahl J B, Kehlet H 1991 Non-steroidal anti-inflammatory drugs: rationale for use in severe post-operative pain. British Journal of Anaesthesia 66: 703–712
Weismann G 1991 Aspirin. Scientific American 264(1): 58–65

6. Intravenous induction agents

THIOPENTONE

Although introduced in 1936, it has remained the standard agent because of its reliability and patient acceptance.

Pharmacokinetics (See Table 6.1)

Distribution

A standard dose of 5 mg/kg given to a 70 kg patient (350 mg, 14 ml of 2.5% solution) over 15 seconds will mix with about 1200 ml of blood (17 heart beats × 70 ml/beat), giving a blood level of about 35 µg/ml of free drug. This profoundly depresses the CNS and also the CVS.

Over the next 3 minutes this will mix with 3800 ml of blood, and some will enter both extracellular and intracellular spaces. Ignoring these, the concentrations will have fallen to 7 µg/ml, 20% of the original level. The drug will begin to leave the vessel-rich group (VRG) of tissues, and awakening (and recovery of blood pressure) will occur. Redistribution to muscle peaks at 20 min, and to fat at about 45 min, further depleting the VRG. The Vd is 1.2–2 l/kg. The t½ of distribution is about 2.5 min., and t½ of redistribution is 45 min.

At 1 min the VRG contains 55% of the dose.

Table 6.1 Pharmacokinetics of intravenous induction agents

	t½β (hours)	Vd (l/kg)	Clearance (ml kg^{-1} min^{-1})	% Protein binding	Infusion rate, (mg kg^{-1} h^{-1})
Thiopentone	8.00–10.00	1.2–2.0	3	75–85	10.0–20.0
Methohexitone	3.00	1.0–2.0	12		3.5–7.0
Propofol	1.25–2.00 (3.00 in the obese)	2.5–10.0	25	98	3.0 (sedation) 6.0 (balanced anaesthesia) 9.0 (sole hypnotic)
Ketamine	2.00–3.00	3.3	20		2.0–4.0
Midazolam	1.70–4.00	1.0–1.8	8	97	0.007–0.014

At 5 min it contains about 25%. The brain content has now fallen to 50% of the 1-minute level.

After 30 min 5% is in the VRG, 75% is in muscle and 18% in fat. The brain content has now fallen by 90%.

After 10 h, of the drug which is not eliminated, 60% is in fat, 35% in muscle and 5% in the VRG.

Haemorrhage reduces blood flow to muscle but perfusion of brain and coronary flow is maintained, and dilution of the dose in blood is proportionately reduced. Hence the effects on the CNS and CVS are enhanced, and dosage must be reduced.

Apprehension increases muscle perfusion so that less of the drug reaches the CNS initially.

Plasma protein binding is high: 75% during induction and 85% when plasma level falls. This prevents the drug coming out of solution in blood (whose pH of 7.4 is much lower than the injected solution which contains 6% sodium carbonate, pH >12; 61% of thiopentone is un-ionized at pH 7.4). Despite the plasma protein binding, spiky crystals of the parent acid have been seen in blood downstream from the injection site, and these almost certainly cause the vascular injury which results from intra-arterial injection (see below).

Impaired renal or hepatic function may result in binding falling to 50%, necessitating a reduction in dosage.

Acute tolerance was thought to occur with thiopentone, with the blood level at arousal being related to the peak blood level during induction, but this has been disproven. Although metabolism is slow, it probably contributes to the early awakening.

Prolonged infusion leads to saturation of muscle and fat. Recovery becomes increasingly dependent on drug metabolism rather than redistribution: after 2 h of infusion, only 20% of the drug is removed from the CNS in the first hour postinfusion.

Elimination

This occurs almost entirely by metabolism. The sulphur atom at C2 is replaced by oxygen, producing pentobarbitone, a long-acting hypnotic. The side-chains at C5 are oxidized and ultimately the ring is opened. 10–15% is metabolized per hour, giving a plasma $t\frac{1}{2}\beta$ of about 10 h.

Only 0.3% is excreted unchanged. The elimination half-life of thiopentone would be *24 years* if renal excretion was the only means of clearance.

Clearance is about 3 ml kg^{-1} min^{-1} (ml/kg per minute) in adults and more than 6 ml kg^{-1} min^{-1} in children, and $t\frac{1}{2}\beta$ is 8–10 h (4–6 h in children), the rate-controlling factor being the return of the drug from the peripheral compartment. Vdss is 1–2 l/kg; 70% of the remaining drug is in the fat at 24 h.

Pharmacodynamics

CNS: Depression is proportional to plasma level: 3–4 mg/kg induces onset of sleep. *Cerebral metabolism and cerebral blood-flow* fall in parallel, by as much as 50%; cerebrovascular resistance may increase by 70%. The EEG alters characteristically. Laryngeal and pharyngeal reflexes tend to increase, so that coughing and laryngeal spasm may follow attempted insertion of an oral airway. Pain perception is increased: some reports suggest that this is an *anti-analgesic effect*, but the matter is controversial as a combination of 0.5 mg/kg of thiopentone and 0.25 mg/kg of propofol has been shown to **raise the pain threshold**. Thiopentone is a potent anticonvulsant in small doses.

CVS: cardiac contractility falls in proportion to the plasma level, with falls in stroke volume and cardiac index. These falls may be further exacerbated by respiratory acidosis. Peripheral vasodilation reduces venous return: there may be a compensatory increase in peripheral vascular resistance. The blood pressure falls, especially in patients with compromised circulation (old age, hypovolaemia, beta-adrenoreceptor block, aortic stenosis, pericardial effusion).

Respiratory system: The respiratory centre is profoundly depressed and sensitivity to CO_2 reduced. When thiopentone is used with an opiate as a total anaesthetic, artificial respiration is mandatory.

Note: in premature infants, postoperative apnoea must be anticipated.

Renal function: renal blood flow falls (but proportionately less than muscle). Release of antidiuretic hormone (enhanced by other drugs, e.g. morphine) leads to oliguria.

Vascular injury occurs because of the chemical nature of the drug (not the alkalinity: a solution of sodium carbonate with the same pH is not injurious). Endothelial damage leads to platelet aggregation and aseptic thrombosis. The vein becomes thickened after 7–10 days in up to 5% of patients, and resolution takes several weeks. **Intra-arterial injection** produces severe pain and thrombosis, followed by ischaemic injury. Although vascular spasm is not a major factor, vasodilators (papaverine and a local anaesthetic) should be injected into the artery before the needle is withdrawn, and heparinization induced to minimize thrombosis in the injured artery. Sympathectomy (local anaesthetic block) should be considered prior to heparinization.

Side-effects

About 8% of patients will move involuntarily, and 4% may cough or have laryngeal spasm. The incidence of these is higher with methohexitone: 33% and 26%. **Immune reactions** are very rare: 1:14000 (methohexitone 1:7000, althesin 1:1000) but are serious, with uncontrollable coughing, bronchospasm and hypotension (see Fig. 3.1).

Contraindications

Respiratory obstruction. Previous immune reaction. Acute intermittent porphyria. Particular care is necessary in: hypovolaemia, septicaemia, severe CVS disease.

METHOHEXITONE (Brietal, Brevital)

An oxybarbiturate (as was hexobarbitone, the first induction barbiturate). A methyl group on the C1 gives excitatory effects in 33% of patients. Both groups on the C5 are unsaturated, leading to faster metabolism than thiopentone. The 1% solution has pH 11, and exposure to CO_2 (in air) results in precipitation of the parent acid, as with thiopentone. At pH 7.4 61% is ionized; plasma protein binding is 70%. Pain at the site of injection is commoner than with thiopentone.

Distribution is similar to thiopentone: Vd is 1–2 l/kg.

Duration to awakening is similar but after-sedation is shorter than with thiopentone due to faster clearance (about 12 ml kg^{-1} min^{-1}), and $t_{1/2}\beta$ is about 3 h.

Note. After-sedation can be detected by a number of tests: Rombergism (standing with eyes closed), placing pegs in matched holes, response to a command, ability to write, simulated motor driving, finding a specified letter in a paragraph of print and a number of tasks requiring attention and mentation.

PROPOFOL (Diprivan)

2:6 di-isopropylphenol, insoluble in water. A 1% solution in an emulsion of soybean oil 1%, egg phosphatide 1.2% and glycerol 2.25%; pH is neutral and solution is isotonic.

Pharmacokinetics

Must be given i.v.. Highly lipophilic: Vd is 2.5–10 l/kg, and highly plasma protein-bound (98%). Initial distribution is similar to thiopentone: $t_{1/2\alpha}$ 2–4 min. Elimination is less than hepatic blood flow, but much faster than thiopentone. Kinetics conform to a three-compartment open model, with clearance from the central compartment at about 25 ml kg^{-1} min^{-1}, and $t_{1/2}\beta$ 16–55 min after a bolus dose. The rapid clearance minimizes the risk of cumulation, and it is suitable for infusion, but prolonged blood sampling reveals a much longer plasma half-life than that after a single dose. This is apparently due to a small fraction which persists in fat, with $t_{1/2}\beta$ 3–6 h, and this may slow recovery after prolonged infusion. Metabolism is by hepatic glucuronide conjugation.

Pharmacodynamics

CNS. Induction in one circulation time, with some euphoria. Central respiratory depression is common. Intracranial pressure and oxygen consumption fall. **Cerebral blood-flow** falls about 25%, and vascular resistance increases by 50%. Recovery on psychomotor testing is rapid but a detectable mild after-effect has been reported. Nausea and vomiting are minimal.

CVS. Centrally-mediated hypotension, especially in hypertensive patients and the elderly. *Cardiac output* falls about 10%, BP by 15% and peripheral vascular resistance by 20%. *Bradycardia* is caused by a central vagotonic action, and may be enhanced by succinylcholine.

Respiratory system: the upper airway muscles are relaxed and reflexes are depressed, facilitating instrumentation.

Local effects: pain on injection is common (30%), especially in small veins. It can be greatly reduced by adding 2 ml 1% lignocaine to 20 ml of the emulsion. Movement is also common. There is no histamine release nor risk of vascular injury, and no risk of tissue damage if the injection is given extravascularly.

Dose

2–2.5 mg/kg <60 years, 1.5 mg/kg >60 years.
Infusion: 3–9 mg kg^{-1} h^{-1}. Blood level : 3–5 μg/ml.
Blood level at consciousness: 1–2.2 μg/ml.

KETAMINE (Ketalar)

A phencyclidine derivative, the hydrochloride being soluble in water.

Pharmacokinetics

Mainly given i.v. (dose 2 mg/kg), but can be given intramuscularly or orally. Elimination is by metabolism with t½β 2–3 h, dependent on liver blood flow. Vdss is 3–8 l/kg, clearance 18 ml kg^{-1} min^{-1}. It is metabolized faster than thiopentone, but the main metabolite, norketamine, is pharmacologically active. Maintenance infusion rate: 2–4 mg kg^{-1} h^{-1} for anaesthesia, 1–2 mg kg^{-1} h^{-1} for analgesia. Although recovery occurs after about 10 min (longer with larger doses), prolonged sedation continues. In this it resembles thiopentone, with its early offset due mainly to redistribution, and a more prolonged period of clearance.

Pharmacodynamics

It appears to block transmission of information from the thalamus to the cortex, resulting in so-called **dissociative anaesthesia**. The eyes may be open and limbs may move, but the patient is unaware and analgesic: painful procedures may be performed (burns dressings) without further anaesthesia. Muscle tone may be increased. Salivary and tracheobronchial secretions are increased, and pharyngeal reflexes depressed: atropine is usually given. Contrary to initial assertions, the airway may become obstructed, and careful monitoring is necessary. **Cerebral blood flow is increased** (this is most probably related to raised CO_2): ketamine is the only i.v. hypnotic which produces this. Blood pressure and intracranial pressure are raised. These sympathomimetic actions are apparently due to CNS stimulation. Hallucinations (auditory, visual and proprioceptive) and confusion occur during awakening in 24–34% of adults (<10% up to 10 years of age) and are more common after atropine or droperidol. They may be suppressed by concurrent dosage with a midazolam 0.05 mg/kg or thiopentone 2 mg/kg.

MIDAZOLAM (Hypnovel, Dormicum)

A benzodiazepine which is water-soluble due to the basic nitrogen in the 2-position of the imidazo ring. The free base is lipophilic.

Pharmacokinetics

Distribution $t\frac{1}{2}$ is 4 min, and $t\frac{1}{2}$ redistribution is 30 min. Elimination $t\frac{1}{2}\beta$ is 1.7–4 h. Plasma level falls by about 90% after 15 min. Kinetics conform to a three-compartment model, with elimination from the central compartment, the rate being dependent on transfer from the peripheral compartments. Clearance is about 5 mg kg^{-1} min^{-1}, the liver extracting about 50%; 97% is plasma protein-bound. Metabolism is to a hydroxy derivative (which is an active drug) and glucuronidation.

Dosage: up to 0.1 mg/kg, and 0.1–0.25 mg kg^{-1} h^{-1} for infusion. Elderly patients may be very susceptible. Midazolam can be given orally as a premedicant, and nasally in children to avoid the unpleasant taste.

Pharmacodynamics

CNS: Profound anterograde amnesia occurs and anxiolysis. Respiratory depression follows doses >0.05 mg/kg. There may be no apparent loss of consciousness, limiting its use as an induction agent: failure to produce sleep may lead to overdose, and it is therefore more suitable as a premedicant. Muscle tone falls. The drug binds to the **specific benzodiazepine receptors,** enhancing the effect of GABA. It is an anticonvulsant. The preparation is non-injurious to veins.

OTHER DRUGS

Fentanyl (Sublimaze)

Although developed as an analgesic, this opioid analgesic has hypnotic properties in higher dosage: 70% of patients are anaesthetized by 30 µg/kg.

Older patients are more susceptible. Muscular rigidity due to effect on spinal neurones is common with high dosage, but is abolished by neuromuscular blockers. Respiratory depression occurs at higher dosage, but cardiovascular stability is retained. Kinetic data are given in Table 5.4.

Sufentanil

A derivative of fentanyl with a rapid onset and shorter elimination half-life (150 min).

   Dose: 0.1–0.2 μg/kg.

Alfentanil

Another related drug also with a rapid onset and short duration (elimination half-life 85–130 min) due to its lower affinity for lipid and smaller volume of distribution.

   Dose: 25–75 μg/kg.

Advantages of narcotic anaesthetics

1. Little cardiac depression.
2. Autoregulation of blood flow to CNS, heart, kidney is unimpaired.
3. Minimal interactions with drugs acting on heart, vessels or autonomics.
4. Intermittent positive pressure ventilation (IPPV) is readily accepted.
5. Endotracheal intubation is tolerated.
6. Prolonged analgesia.
7. Absence of toxic effects on liver and kidney.
8. Can be antagonized if necessary.
9. Effective during cardiopulmonary bypass (lungs out of circuit, difficulty administering volatile agents.)

Alphadione (Althesin)

A mixture of two steroids, *alphaxalone* (a potent but insoluble hypnotic) and *alphadolone* (a solubilizer), dissolved in polyoxyethylated castor oil (Cremophor EL). Severe immune reactions related to the vehicle severely restricted the use of this agent although it was an effective hypnotic with rapid metabolism (unless the elimination route was saturated by high dosage). Involuntary movements occurred during induction.

   Historical note: An earlier derivative of the pregnane-dione nucleus was *hydroxydione* (Viadril). It became obsolete because of venous injury, very high cost and prolonged action.

Etomidate (Hypnomidate)

An imidazole derivative. A dose of 0.2–0.3 mg/kg induces loss of consciousness within 65 seconds. The drug is rapidly hydrolysed by esterases in the plasma and liver. Arousal occurs in about 6 min. It causes less depression of the cardiovascular system than thiopentone, making this agent particularly useful in haemodynamically compromised patients. There is a higher incidence of involuntary movements, pain on injection and nausea than after thiopentone. As a sedative in the intensive care unit (ICU) it was found to specifically inhibit cortisol production from II-deoxycortisol.

Gamma hydroxy-butyrate (Gamma-OH)

A close relative to GABA, the CNS transmitter, a dose of 50–70 mg/kg takes 3–5 min to induce sleep of prolonged duration. Involuntary movements are common, as is postanaesthetic vomiting. Up to 10% of patients awake with hallucinations. An obsolete agent.

Propanidid (Epontol)

An ester of eugenol, the only i.v. hypnotic to be rapidly metabolized (by plasma cholinesterase). Its very short half-life was advantageous, but side-effects limited its usefulness. Now also obsolete.

GENERAL COMMENT ON INTRAVENOUS HYPNOTICS

Except for ketamine and the narcotic anaesthetics, these drugs are **not general anaesthetics:** they do not produce analgesia and depression of reflex response to pain except at doses which profoundly depress the CNS and cardiovascular system.

The standard with which new drugs should be compared is thiopentone. Although it has been in use since 1936, its high patient acceptability, reliability, relative freedom from side-effects and economy have enabled it to retain a premier role despite repeated attempts at synthesizing drugs to replace it. It is interesting to note that when it was first introduced there was unacceptable morbidity and mortality due to overdose and lack of appreciation of its limitations as an anaesthetic.

7. Inhalation anaesthetics

THE IDEAL INHALATIONAL ANAESTHETIC

1. *Low solubility:* hence

   - rapid onset
   - rapid offset
   - depth readily alterable.

2. *Easily administered:*

   - simple apparatus
   - not irritating to the airways
   - high safety margin.

3. *Minimal side-effects.*
4. *Minimal toxicity.*
5. *Minimal metabolism.*
6. *Safe in all age groups.*
7. *High potency*, enabling it to be given with high FiO_2. (FiO_2 is the percentage of oxygen in the inhaled gas mixture converted to a fraction, e.g. 50% is 0.5.)
8. *Analgesic*
9. *Chemically stable:*

   - long shelf-life
   - not affected by light and oxygen
   - compatible with soda-lime
   - compatible with metals and plastics of anaesthetic apparatus.

10. *No environmental hazard:*

    - in trace concentrations, to operating room staff
    - when vented to the atmosphere.

11. *Not prone to cause **cardiac arrhythmias** with catecholamines*
12. *Not inflammable with oxygen-enriched gas mixtures*
13. *Favourable physical characteristics:*

- boiling point above ambient temperatures enables simple storage, and use in vaporizers
- low latent heat of vaporization simplifies vaporizer design.

The mode of action of anaesthetics is discussed in Chapter 2.

TOXICITY

The first inhalational anaesthetic recognized to be toxic was chloroform (i.e hepatotoxic). Intrinsic toxicity was thought to be uncommon until it was found that most anaesthetics undergo metabolism and some metabolites are toxic. Up to 75% of methoxyflurane may be biotransformed, with release of fluoride ion. A serum level of 50 mmol/l (millimoles/litre) of fluoride ions injures the renal tubular cells, producing polyuric renal failure: a limit of 2.5 MAC-hours was imposed (except in children who store fluoride in bone). With enflurane 3% is metabolized, but free fluoride levels do not reach toxic levels until after 9.6 MAC-hours.

The metabolism of **halothane** has been the subject of controversy and study, due to the occasional occurrence of halothane toxicity. The *National Halothane Study* (from the USA) reported an incidence of halothane hepatitis as 1:35 000 anaesthetics. Of reported cases, 85% had had multiple halothane anaesthetics, the last usually within a month, and 33% had had an unexplained fever following a previous halothane anaesthetic. The onset was earliest in those who had had repeated exposures: 6–11 days after one and 3–6 days after repeated anaesthetics. Early onset was related to severity, as was jaundice. A total of 75% presented with fever; 50% had anorexia, nausea and vomiting; 30% had eosinophilia; 10% had skin rash, and some also had joint pains. Liver failure caused death in 20–50% of patients. Adverse prognostic factors were age over 40 years, prothrombin time over 40 seconds, obesity, and serum bilirubin exceeding 200 μmol/l. The majority of cases were obese and 70% of cases were female. Children have been subsequently reported as being less susceptible. Three possible mechanisms have been proposed:

a. *Reductive metabolism* producing an unpaired covalent electron in a highly reactive radical. This causes lipid peroxidation to long-chain fatty acids, injuring the cell directly or by an immune mechanism.

b. *An immune response,* as surviving patients have been found to have an antibody which reacts with halothane-exposed rabbit hepatocytes.

There is evidence that metabolites of inhaled vapours can bind covalently to liver protein, producing an antigen. Immune-based liver toxicity would then be related to the amount of metabolism, with the risk being halothane > enflurane > isoflurane.

c. *Depression of the immune response,* especially in those incubating viral hepatitis, producing the acute disease which is histologically indistinguishable from halothane hepatitis.

MAC

The **minimum alveolar anaesthetic concentration** needed to suppress reflex movement in response to a standard surgical stimulus (incision on the forearm) in 50% of subjects.

MAC enables accurate comparisons to be made between inhalation anaesthetics, and is a guide for the clinical use of these drugs.

MAC varies with age. For halothane it is 0.76% between 31 and 55 years, but 1.06% up to 6 months of age, and 0.64% at 70 years.

MAC is decreased with the concomitant use of other hypnotics e.g. premedicants or narcotic analgesics. For inhalation anaesthetic mixtures it is additive. The MAC of a volatile anaesthetic is decreased by 1% for each 1% of nitrous oxide in the gas mixture, MAC of N_2O being 105%. It is also reduced by 30% with morphine 0.15 mg/kg.

Pharmacodynamics of inhalation anaesthetics

CNS. Progressive depression of normal function occurs in the cortex, basal ganglia, cerebellum, spinal sensory, spinal motor, respiratory centres and vasomotor centre. Loss of higher inhibitory centres may unmask excitatory activity (delirium, laryngeal spasm). Enflurane produces EEG spikes characteristics of convulsive activity in deeper levels.

Autonomic nervous system. Generally depression occurs, but there may be imbalance, e.g. vagotonic slowing of the heart with halothane.

CVS. Myocardial contractility is progressively depressed: enflurane > halothane > isoflurane. Myocardial irritability with catecholamines is increased with halogenated agents: halothane > ethers (enflurane, isoflurane), an effect increased by respiratory acidosis.

  Blood pressure falls with increasing depth: enflurane > halothane > isoflurane. *Cardiac output* falls with increasing depth: perfusion to the brain and heart is sustained by reducing that to the liver, gut, kidneys and skin.

Respiratory system. Rate and depth of ventilation decrease: with spontaneous respiration, alveolar CO_2 rises as depth of ventilation decreases. Functional residual capacity falls, and ventilation/perfusion mismatch increases. **Increased FiO_2 is obligatory.**

Skeletal muscle. Muscle tone falls but direct depression of the neuromuscular junction (NMJ) occurs only with deep anaesthesia.

Renal function. Renal blood flow falls with decreased glomerular filtration. Antidiuretic hormone release is increased with concomitant drugs, leading to oliguria.

Liver function. Blood flow and metabolic activity fall with deep anaesthesia, effects enhanced by reduced blood pressure or a fall in arterial oxygen saturation.

Temperature control. Regulation is depressed with heat loss increased due to skin vasodilation.

Operating room pollution

Following a report of increased incidence of miscarriage in theatre staff, extensive studies have been conducted into the risk of inhaling trace amounts of anaesthetic gases, and several types of extracting devices have been devised to remove the exhaled gases. It is interesting to note that the data is insufficient to indicate a risk even at the $p = 0.1$ level for any hazard other than miscarriage, and further controlled studies are precluded by industrial environmental legislation.

Pharmacokinetics of inhaled anaesthetics

See Section 1:1.

NITROUS OXIDE, N_2O

Manufacture

Ammonium nitrate decomposes when heated:

$$NH_4NO_3 \rightarrow N_2O + 2H_2O$$

The gas is thoroughly dried, and the impurities are then nitrogen (which is a harmless diluent), and higher oxides of nitrogen: nitric oxide (NO which spontaneously oxidizes to dinitrogen tetraoxide N_2O_4) which then reacts with water to form nitrous and nitric acids:

$$N_2O_4 + H_2O \rightarrow HNO_2 + HNO_3$$

These cause acute chemical pneumonitis.

Pharmacokinetics

The MAC is 105%, so that a high alveolar concentration and a volatile supplement are necessary. A high alveolar P_{N_2O} can be obtained (at sea level) only by removing nitrogen from the alveolar gas, as the alveolar pressures of oxygen (100 mm), CO_2 (40 mm) and water vapour (46 mm) are fixed, and Dalton's Law requires that the sum of the pressures is about 760 mm. **Nitrogen washout** requires a high flow of fresh gases initially. The **3,4,5 rule** is helpful: after 3 minutes breathing into a circuit with 4 litres fresh gas flow the end-expired nitrogen is less than 5% (with normal V/Q ratio of 0.8).

N_2O is more soluble in blood (0.47 ml/ml blood) than nitrogen is (0.014 ml/ml). During induction it enters blood faster than N_2 leaves it, and during emergence it leaves faster than N_2 enters. Three observed effects arise from this:

1. *Second gas effect.* When a volatile agent and N_2O are given, the rapid absorption of N_2O results in a rise of partial pressure of the volatile vapour, enhancing its rate of uptake.

2. *Concentration effect.* When a high concentration of N_2O (75%) is given, its initial rapid absorption from the alveoli results in a fall of alveolar pressure. Further N_2O/O_2 is drawn into the alveoli, *increasing the amount of N_2O available without increasing the alveolar ventilation.*

3. *Diffusion hypoxia.* Transient cyanosis may occur during emergence from N_2O if respiration is depressed. This is due to the inhalation of air (21% O_2) which is diluted by the rapid excretion of N_2O, N_2 being absorbed only slowly. The phenomenon is seen only when alveolar ventilation is depressed, and is avoided by enriching the inspired FiO_2 at the completion of anaesthesia and during recovery.

Pharmacodynamics

Rapid and reversible depression of the *CNS*. Analgesia occurs early: 30% N_2O is used for **relative analgesia** in dentistry and for wound dressings, and 50–70% with oxygen in obstetrics.

It is a weak *cardiac depressant*, the effect being compensated by mild sympathetic stimulation. If the latter is suppressed by concomitant drugs, the hypotensive effect may be unmasked. It increases pulmonary vascular resistance in the neonate. It is reported to produce nausea by action on endogenous opiate receptors. It also diffuses into any gas-containing spaces (e.g. middle ear, bowel) and causes unwanted distension.

Disadvantages

It is *cumbersome* to provide in remote areas as it is contained in cylinders. It requires special apparatus to deliver a safe mixture and to economize in its consumption. At altitude the reduced atmospheric pressure requires greater supplementation with a volatile vapour.

Bone marrow depression. It depresses methionine synthetase, with corresponding depression of deoxythymidine synthesis and cell replication. Rapidly dividing cells are most affected, especially leucocytes and erythrocytes. It is hazardous only with prolonged or repeated exposure or in very ill patients.

Gas-containing cavities will expand as N_2O enters faster than N_2 leaves. The expansion may embarrass respiration (lung cysts), stress suture lines (bowel gas), lift a graft off the ear drum or overdistend the cuff of an endotracheal tube. The effect is reversed during recovery.

HALOTHANE

The first widely applicable non-inflammable vapour. Introduced by ICI in 1956 after development by Raventos.

Chemistry

Bromochlorotrifluoroethane, a 2-carbon molecule that is not an ether. Difficult to synthesize compared with its predecessors. Stabilized with 0.01% thymol which does not volatilize and thus accumulates in the vaporizer.

Not flammable in air or oxygen. Boiling point 50 °C. Vapour pressure 32 kPa (241 mm) at 20 °C.

Pharmacokinetics

Moderate solubility in blood (blood–gas partition coefficient = 2.3) and brain (grey matter–blood partition coefficient = 2.1) gives fast induction. Tissues equilibrate quickly except fat (fat–blood coefficient = 60) which takes days. Inhaled concentration must be kept above MAC for some time. During recovery halothane is excreted by the lungs but also continues to enter the fat, with faster awakening than would be predicted from blood/gas solubility. If fat is moderately saturated by prolonged anaesthesia, recovery is markedly slowed.

Pharmacodynamics

CNS. Rapid loss of consciousness without excitement. Respiratory depression occurs early, with raised end-tidal CO_2, especially if opioids or other central depressants are used. A weak analgesic compared with the ethers. Cerebral blood flow and intracranial pressure increase, especially if CO_2 retention occurs. Vomiting is rare.

The *sympathetic nervous system* is depressed: falls in blood pressure are readily induced. Vagal tone persists, giving a bradycardia unless atropine is used.

The *ventilatory response* to hypoxia is impaired: routine use of oxygen during the recovery period is strongly recommended.

CVS. Hypotension readily occurs due to depression of the myocardium, medullary centres, sympathetic ganglia and vascular smooth muscle. The SA node and AV conduction are also depressed. Blood pressure tends to recover during longer exposures. **Cardiac arrhythmias** are readily provoked by catecholamines, especially if CO_2 retention and hypoxia also occur. Adrenaline dosage should not exceed 1–2 µg/kg. If arrhythmias occur, lignocaine or a beta-adrenoreceptor blocker (propranolol, or metoprolol in asthmatics) should be given.

Respiratory system. Minimal bronchial irritation and bronchial dilation occur. Hypoxic pulmonary vasoconstriction is impaired.

Skeletal muscle. Contractility is reduced (20% at 1.5 × MAC), enhancing neuromuscular block. *Halothane tremors* (shakes) are common during recovery, especially with longer anaesthetics: they appear to be related to a disturbance of Ca^{2+} release and re-uptake by the sarcoplasmic reticulum as they appear as muscle tone returns.

Uterus. Contractility is severely impaired by inspired concentrations greater than 0.5%.

Final comment

Despite its disadvantages, halothane is still a very useful agent. Its lack of irritation and potency make it a particularly good agent for inhalational inductions. It is not contraindicated in biliary obstruction despite its occasional hepatotoxicity. Controversy exists about its use with spontaneous respiration during long cases, due to the hypercarbia that occurs.

ENFLURANE (Ethrane)

Chemistry

$CHFCl-CF_2-O-CF_2H$: an ethylmethyl ether. Boiling point is 57 °C, vapour pressure 23 kPa (170 mm). Non-inflammable.

Pharmacokinetics

Blood–gas solubility 1.9, giving fast induction and recovery. Relatively high MAC (1.54%) but inspired vapour is well tolerated. Fat solubility is lower than with halothane, shortening the time to equilibration.

Metabolism. A small proportion is broken down, with release of fluoride ion from the alpha-carbon. Reported levels of 15–20 µmol/l are below those hazardous to renal tubules (50 µmol/l).

Pharmacodynamics

CNS metabolism and bloodflow are reduced. Analgesia occurs. The **EEG** is unusual in that with deep anaesthesia (3–4%) the characteristic high-voltage slow waves are interrupted by periods of electrical silence punctuated by spike activity similar to that seen during convulsions: muscle twitches may occur. Hypocarbia ($PaCO_2$ 20 mm) increases the amount of spiking. Experience has shown that this effect is not clinically important, except in epileptic patients.

Respiratory system. Response to CO_2 is depressed: *raised end-tidal CO_2* occurs during spontaneous respiration.

CVS: hypotension is readily produced. Heart rate and rhythm are stable, and more resistant to arrhythmias with catecholamines than with halothane. Systemic peripheral resistance falls by 25%, more than with other inhalation agents.

Skeletal muscle. Non-depolarizing blockers are enhanced: dosage may be reduced 30–50%. Diethyl ether has a similar effect.

Comment

Enflurane is a safe alternative to halothane as hepatic necrosis has been reported only rarely. It is well tolerated and gives easy control of blood pressure. Awakening is rapid. It is relatively expensive, leading to its use mainly in low-flow circuits.

ISOFLURANE

Chemistry

$CF_3CHCl-O-CF_2H$: a methylethyl ether, an isomer of enflurane. The lack of fluorine on the 1-carbon results in no fluoride ion being released by metabolism.

Pharmacokinetics

Low blood–gas partition coefficient (1.3) and low MAC (1.15%) enable rapid induction and recovery to be achieved. Fat solubility similar to enflurane, with earlier equilibration than halothane.

Metabolism is minimal, due to the stability of the 2-carbon–fluorine bonds.

Pharmacodynamics

CNS. It is analgesic. The rise in intracranial pressure is smaller than with other volatile agents, making it the agent of choice in neuroanaesthesia.

Respiratory control is depressed: end-tidal PCO_2 rises with spontaneous respiration. It is mildly irritant to the airways. Laryngospasm is more commonly seen than with halothane.

CVS. The systemic vascular resistance falls significantly. Baroreflex activity is retained, the resulting tachycardia may cause a rise in cardiac output. Rhythm is stable and resistant to effects of catecholamines. Isoflurane has been implicated with 'coronary artery steal'. This is not clinically significant if the diastolic blood pressure is maintained.

Skeletal muscle. Non-depolarizing blockers are enhanced as with enflurane.

Uterus is relaxed.

Comment

Circulatory stability is a leading feature of isoflurane. It is a useful adjunct to induce hypotension. Respiratory depression limits its usefulness with spontaneous respiration. It is considered to be the least likely agent to cause hepatotoxicity. It is used mainly in low-flow circuits due to its cost.

DESFLURANE (Jones 1990)

An ethylmethyl ether similar to isoflurane, but with fluorine on the 1-carbon. It is less potent (MAC 6%) than isoflurane, and volatile, with boiling point 23.5 °C, vapour pressure 58.5 kPa (439 mm) and would need special vaporizing apparatus. Blood–gas partition coefficient is very low (0.5) as is the fat–blood partition (27, isoflurane is 45), making induction and elimination similar to nitrous oxide (blood–gas coefficient 0.47). The respiratory effects and cardiovascular actions are similar to isoflurane, and metabolism is minimal. Current data indicate a useful role in anaesthesia.

SEVOFLURANE (Jones 1990)

A halogenated methylisopropyl ether; MAC is 2%, boiling point 58.5 °C and vapour pressure 21 kPa (157 mm) at 20 °C. Blood–gas partition is also very low at 0.6, and the fat–blood partition coefficient is 48 (isoflurane: 45), making induction and elimination rapid. It is unstable with warm soda-lime, a property which would limit its usefulness.

METHOXYFLURANE

Chemistry

The first of the halogenated ethers 1,1,difluro, 2,2,dichloro-ethyl methyl ether. Non-flammable.

Pharmacokinetics

High blood–gas (11) and fat–blood (61) partition coefficients, and very soluble in rubber (630). High boiling point (105 °C) with low vapour pressure (24 mm) make induction slow despite very low MAC (0.16%) and recovery is very prolonged.

Metabolism. Extensively metabolized with fluoride released from 1-carbon. After 2.5 MAC-hours, fluoride level rises to 50 µmol/l, a level which injures renal tubules, leading to polyuric renal failure: children are more tolerant as they sequester F^- in their rapidly growing bones. Methoxyflurane induces enzymes, increasing metabolism of many drugs (including itself). With tetracycline drugs, an alternative pathway produces oxalate as a metabolite, with the risk of oxalic acid crystalluria in the renal tubules.

DIETHYL ETHER

Chemistry

C_2H_5-O-C_2H_5. Its historical importance is greater than its use. Easily prepared and stored. Highly flammable in air or O_2.

Pharmacokinetics

Very soluble: partition coefficients blood–gas 12, fat–blood 73. MAC 1.9%, boiling point 35 °C. Hence readily vaporizable (vapour pressure 440 mm at

20 °C), but irritant to airways and induction slow. Its solubility also makes emergence slow.

Metabolism is substantial, with metabolites harmless as they enter the Krebs cycle.

Pharmacodynamics

Respiratory depression is masked by release of catecholamines consequent on the irritation of the airways so that simple inhalation anaesthesia is safe. Circulatory depression also occurs late due to the catecholamine release, but in the absence of the latter or with adrenergic blocking drugs, profound depression occurs. The catecholamine release also results in bronchodilation: ether has been used therapeutically in bronchial asthma. Secretions are stimulated, and anticholinergic premedication essential. Prolonged nausea and vomiting are common: this effect and its flammability led to ether's rapid decline when halothane was introduced in 1956. Uterine tone is only slightly depressed in light anaesthesia. Skeletal tone is progressively depressed, a property which made ether suitable for a wide range of surgery before neuromuscular blockers became available. It greatly enhances non-depolarizing block.

TRICHLORETHYLENE

Chemistry

$CCl_2 = CHCl$, an unsaturated olefin, also used in dry cleaning. After chloroform, the first non-flammable halogenated agent. Easily made and stored and is very cheap. **Unstable with warm soda-lime:** dichloracetylene, C_2Cl_2, a potent nerve poison, is produced, a major factor in its decline in popularity.

Pharmacokinetics

Very soluble in blood (blood–gas coefficient 9.1) and fat (fat–blood coefficient 107). Its very low MAC (0.17%) makes it usable despite its low volatility (boiling point 87 °C) and its irritant effect on the airways, but induction is very slow as is recovery.

Metabolism. Much is metabolized to trichlorethanol, a long-acting sedative, making recovery even slower after prolonged use.

Pharmacodynamics

A very good analgesic. It produces rapid, shallow respiration with CO_2 retention, and is suitable only for brief inhalation anaesthesia with spontaneous respiration. The heart is sensitized to catecholamines, especially with the respiratory acidosis which readily occurs. Skeletal and uterine muscle are poorly relaxed.

CYCLOPROPANE

Pharmacokinetics

It is a gas at 20 °C, and compressed into a liquid at 6.5 atmospheres pressure. Blood–gas solubility is 0.42, similar to N_2O. Fat–gas solubility is high (15), and MAC is also high (9.2%). Induction with a high inspired fraction (50% in oxygen) is rapid, but equilibration is slow. Recovery is fast only after a brief anaesthetic. It is not metabolized, the cyclic structure being very stable. Explosive in air or oxygen.

Pharmacodynamics

It is a good analgesic. Respiratory depression occurs with increasing depth: cyclopropane apnoea was used during intermittent positive pressure respiration (IPPR) prior to muscle relaxants. It produces the release of catecholamines, with maintenance of blood pressure but susceptibility to arrhythmias due to increased irritability of the myocardium (and hypercarbia with spontaneous respiration). These effects and its flammability have led to its decline but it is still used as an induction agent in paediatrics.

FURTHER READING

Jones R M 1990 Desflurane and sevoflurane: inhalation agents for this decade? British Journal of Anaesthesia 65: 527–536
National Halothane Study 1966 Possible association between halothane anesthesia and postoperative liver necrosis. Journal of the American Medical Association 197: 775–788

8. The neuromuscular junction

THE MOTOR UNIT

This comprises a motor neurone (mainly in the anterior horn of the cord), a motor axon (A-alpha fibre, conducting at 80–120 m/s) and the muscle fibres supplied by it. The neurone may branch to supply several fibres: the larger and stronger the muscle and the coarser its movement, the greater the branching e.g. gluteal muscles. In contrast, external eye muscles subserve very fine movements (saccadic) so that the ratio of muscle fibres to neurones is almost one.

The nerve axons terminate as *end-plates* which lie in gutters in the muscle fibres: in long fibres there are multiple end-plates to ensure that contraction is synchronous.

In *old age* the number of end-plates decreases, with a loss of tone and power in the muscles and a corresponding decrease in the dose of muscle relaxants.

MUSCLE TONE

The *myotatic reflex* of the spinal cord, modified by higher centres, maintains tension in a muscle by contraction of alternating groups of fibres (to prevent fatigue) to maintain posture. The **muscle spindle** also maintains tone by matching the length of the muscle to the distance between its origin and insertion, so the muscle is ready to respond to a stimulus without having to 'take up the slack'. Skeletal muscles are never flaccid except in deep sleep or when reflexes are depressed as in anaesthesia.

The muscle spindle has a small muscle fibre at each end innervated by a gamma-efferent motor neurone (conduction velocity 30–70 m/s). Between the fibres are nuclear bag elements (nuclei grouped in the middle) responding to length, and nuclear chain elements (nuclei strung out) responding to tension: annulospiral nerve endings innervate both elements, and A fibres carry afferent impulses at 30–70 m/s to the posterior horn. If the surrounding muscle contracts and shortens, the spindle senses this and reflexively contracts its motor fibres to match its length to the surrounding muscle. If the muscle is stretched by a load, the spindle reflexively increases the contraction of the parent muscle to match the load. The spindle provides **positive**

feedback, enabling the parent muscle to maintain a set length and tension unless over-ruled by higher centres. During anaesthesia, muscle tone maintained by the spindles interferes with access to the abdominal viscera unless inhibited by deep anaesthesia or by neuromuscular blocking drugs (which may also block the gamma-efferent neurone end-plates).

During light sleep with thiopentone, tone is preserved and muscles can respond reflexively to painful stimuli. With high doses the response is lessened, and tone is also impaired with a risk of airway obstruction.

NEUROMUSCULAR TRANSMISSION

Acetylcholine (ACh) is synthesized from choline and acetyl coenzyme A by choline acetyl transferase in the nerve ending. The enzyme diffuses from the neurone down the axon. Choline enters through the cell membrane: its entry can be blocked by hemicholinium (experimentally) resulting in depletion of the ACh. ACh is stored in vesicles which are small sections of infolded cell membrane nipped off to form spheres of 50 nm radius.

ACh is also a transmitter in the CNS, all preganglionic autonomic synapses (nicotinic) and postganglionic cholinergic sites (muscarinic – mainly para-sympathetic).

Miniature end-plate potentials occur at the neuromuscular junction (NMJ) from the random release of ACh from vesicles, but do not evoke a muscle response. They appear to have a role in regulating the sensitivity of the junction to ACh by maintaining integrity of the ACh receptors (which are constantly being renewed), as a spreading of ACh receptors over the muscle membrane and altered response to ACh (and succinylcholine) is seen from 3 days after denervation.

Excitation–secretion coupling

The arrival of a nerve impulse activates *adenyl cyclase* which converts ATP to cyclic 3:5 adenosine monophosphate *(cAMP)*. This activates **protein kinase** which phosphorylates proteins which control several functions of the nerve ending including Ca^{2+} **entry and ACh release.** Phosphodiesterase inactivates the cAMP.

An antagonist to cAMP has been synthesized and inhibits this series of responses, but has not been used in anaesthesia. *Phosphodiesterase inhibitors* (azathioprine, aminophylline, high-dosage frusemide) enhance transmission, and adenylate cyclase inhibitors (low-dosage frusemide or alloxan) depress it. *Amrinone and milrinone* are *phosphodiesterase-III inhibitors* but act only on smooth and cardiac muscle.

A single stimulus releases about 100 vesicles of ACh (in intercostal muscle) with 10^4 molecules of ACh per vesicle. *Repetitive stimuli* (a tetanus) result in a fall in the number of vesicles released: 82 per impulse at 5 Hz, 62 per impulse at 50 Hz, and correspondingly less ACh. This decline forms the basis for tests of non-depolarizing block (see below). There are about 500 vesicles available for release, and they are mobilized in the nerve ending to the site of release at the rate of 2500 per second. The wall of the vesicle fuses with the cell membrane, thus completing the cycle of infolding, pinching off, migrating and rejoining.

Ca^{2+} is associated with the **mobilization of vesicles** so they aggregate in triangular groups opposite the 'shoulders' of the clefts in the opposing postjunctional membrane.

During stimulation the synthesis of ACh increases under the influence of presynaptic receptors (see presynaptic augmentation, below). At the same time the number of vesicles near the clefts falls, so that the amount of *ACh released per stimulus falls* until an equilibrium is reached. When stimulation ceases vesicular ACh increases so the *next stimulus releases more ACh than normal.* The process of depletion underlies the 'train-of-four' test for neuromuscular (NM) block: the decreasing release of ACh with repetitive stimuli results in *'fade'* because of the competitive nature of the block: the less ACh present, the more effective the non-depolarizing blocking drug becomes. When repetitive stimulation stops for a few seconds the ACh vesicles increase, and the first 'posttetanic' stimulus produces an increased release and a supranormal response: *posttetanic facilitation.*

Presynaptic augmentation of ACh release

Presynaptic receptors on the nerve ending are acted on by ACh, enhancing the production and mobilization of ACh – an example of positive feedback. These receptors are blocked by d-tubocurarine and metocurine, enhancing block further. Pancuronium and vecuronium appear to act only post synaptically. Alpha-bungarotoxin irreversibly blocks postsynaptic receptors, revealing presynaptic block experimentally.

TESTS FOR NEUROMUSCULAR BLOCK

Repetitive stimuli lead to a *depletion* of ACh in the nerve ending, so that the amount released per stimulus falls to a lower but steady level. As ACh *competes* with non-depolarizing blockers for the postjunctional receptors, **the falling amount of ACh released per stimulus will be apparent as increased block.**

Train-of-four testing uses four supramaximal stimuli applied to the ulnar nerve at the wrist at 0.5 s intervals (see Fig. 8.1). The normal muscle responds with four equal twitches (of the adductor pollicis) which may be measured visually, mechanically or electrically. As non-depolarizing block occurs the falling ACh release with repeated stimuli leads to a falling response, and the ratio of the fourth to the first response is the *train-of-four* (T4) *ratio*. A T4 ratio of 0.7 or more is desirable before the patient is allowed to resume spontaneous breathing.

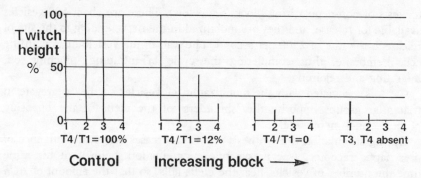

Fig. 8.1 Train-of-four. Increasing block progressively decreases the size of the twitches, with disappearance of the 4th, then the third, the 2nd and ultimately the 1st.

Double-burst stimulation employs the same principle: two short bursts (about 3 stimuli each) at 50 Hz separated by 0.75 s produce two contractions, the second being smaller. This allows a better appreciation of the degree of fade when the twitch sizes are compared manually.

Posttetanic count (PTC) depends on the increased mobilization of ACh in the nerve ending which occurs with repeated stimulation. A repetitive stimulation (tetanus) at 50 Hz is applied for 5 s. After a short pause, single stimuli are applied each second, and the number of responses counted (the PTC). This response is still detectable at deep levels of paralysis when single twitches have almost disappeared. Even at 1 Hz the ACh becomes depleted, resulting in a limited number of responses in proportion to the block. The increased response which follows a pause after previous stimulation is termed **posttetanic facilitation**.

THE NEUROMUSCULAR JUNCTION (See Fig. 8.2)

There are 2–4 million receptors per junction, a large excess over the number needed to effect transmission. There is thus a **margin of safety** (see Table 8.1): no impairment of conduction occurs until most of the receptors are blocked.

Cholinesterase is present in abundance in the cleft. It hydrolyses 60% of ACh before the transmitter can reach the receptors: hence an **anticholinesterase** will allow more ACh to reach the receptors and compete with non-depolarizing blockers. All the ACh is hydrolysed in 1 millisecond (ms) allowing physiological stimulation rates up to 100 Hz. Each hydrolytic site on cholinesterase removes 10^6 ACh molecules per second. Clinical doses of anticholinesterase (0.05–0.1 mg neostigmine/kg) inhibit only part of the cholinesterase, allowing more of the ACh to reach the receptors, but not preventing rapid hydrolysis. If more complete inhibition is achieved, depolarizing or **cholinergic block** will result, similar to that seen with suxamethonium.

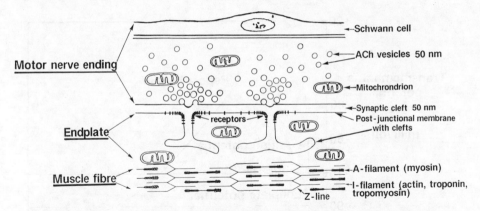

Fig. 8.2 The neuromuscular junction (diagrammatic). The nerve lies in a gutter of the muscle membrane, separated by about 50 nm. The membrane is altered adjacent to the nerve, being extensively folded, with multiple clefts: the 'postjunctional membrane (PJM)' or 'end-plate'. The vesicles of ACh are aggregated into triangular groups opposite the clefts, and the ACh receptors are grouped on the shoulders of the clefts.

Table 8.1 Margin of safety

Stimulation rate (Hz)	% of receptors needed for response	Observations
1	15–20	Normal twitch
30	30	
50	40	Train-of-four ratio 0.7
100	50	Sustained tetanus
200	66	Sustained head lift

POSTJUNCTIONAL MEMBRANE (End-plate)

The muscle membrane adjacent to the nerve becomes modified, increasing its sensitivity to ACh 1000-fold by developing clefts and large numbers of receptors. The change is acquired, as muscle is mesoderm and nerves ectoderm, and new end-plates can be formed during life.

Receptors are grouped on the shoulders of the clefts. They undergo constant degeneration and replacement, their t½ varying from 18 h to weeks (depending on the level of activity: they last longer when active). In *myasthenia gravis* a circulating antibody to receptor protein reduces their number to 30% of normal, with impairment of transmission and profound sensitivity to non-depolarizing blockers.

Each receptor site has 5 subunits, two being alpha units with molecular weight of 40 000 daltons. These must both be actuated to open the ion channel (by twisting the circular pattern of the units), allowing the entry of Na^+ and Ca^{2+} and exit of K^+. The extracellular part of the channel is wider,

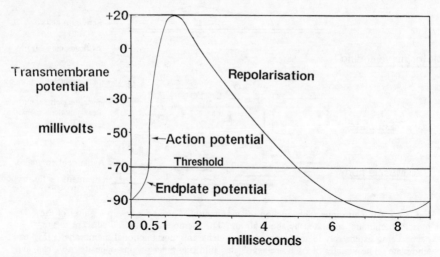

Fig. 8.3   End-plate and action potentials. See text for explanation.

making it cone-shaped. Some drugs that have large molecules enter the channel and obstruct the passage of ions giving open-channel block, others can occlude the entry giving closed-channel block.

The membrane is **polarized** with the inside about 90 mv negative. ACh results in depolarization: an **end-plate potential** (EPP, see Fig. 8.3). The ACh in each vesicle opens 2000 channels: 100 vesicles thus open 200 000 channels, with the entry of 3×10^9 Na$^+$ ions. When the EPP reaches about -70 mv, the depolarization is propagated to the remainder of the muscle fibre, producing an **action potential** (see Fig 8.3 also). The electrical changes are complete in about 10 ms, after which muscle contraction occurs, and the junction is ready for the next stimulus.

EXCITATION–CONTRACTION COUPLING

Depolarization spreads from the end-plate over the muscle, enters the transverse tubular system and reaches the longitudinal tubular system (*sarcoplasmic reticulum*). Ca^{2+} ions are released, the process of shortening occurs and Ca^{2+} is pumped back into the reticulum, allowing the muscle to relax.

Ca^{2+} release is greatly increased by suxamethonium, and its re-uptake slowed by halothane. As the tonic form of malignant hyperpyrexia is associated with abnormal re-uptake of Ca^{2+}, the role of these drugs in initiating the syndrome is explained. **Dantrolene** reduces Ca^{2+} release from the reticulum, hence its therapeutic use in hyperpyrexia.

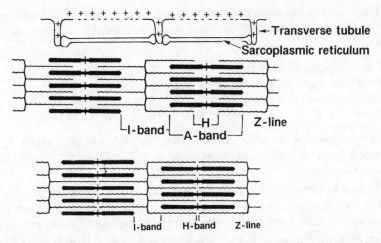

Fig. 8.4 Muscle structure. The A-band is seen where the H-band (myosin) overlaps the I-band (actin).

MUSCLE CONTRACTION

Myosin, the thicker fibre, forms a charged intermediate which binds with *actin*, the thin fibre (see Fig. 8.4). The cross-bridges formed then swivel, propelling the actin filament along the myosin and shortening the fibre. ATP provides the energy for this. The cross-bridging is inhibited by *tropomyosin* which is wrapped around the actin helix. Tropomyosin is stabilized by *troponin*, a globular protein. Ca^{2+} acts by attaching to the troponin, which in turn alters the tropomyosin inhibition and allows the actin–myosin cross-bridges to form. Energy (as ATP) is required to maintain the muscle in a relaxed state. When deprived of nutrients and oxygen (as in cramp or rigor mortis), the muscle remains contracted. *ATP provides the energy*, complexing with myosin and converting to ADP; and Ca^{2+} *controls the process.*

CHOLINESTERASE

There are two types of cholinesterase:

1. *True or acetylcholinesterase,* found in cells especially the brain, erythrocytes and neuromuscular junction.
2. *Pseudo- or plasma or butyrylcholinesterase.* Plasma cholinesterase has no normal function, and if it is abnormal or absent it remains undetected unless the patient is given drugs which are metabolized by it e.g. suxamethonium, procaine, atracurium: the actions of these are prolonged.

In 1949 Bovet-Nitti observed that suxamethonium is hydrolysed by plasma cholinesterase, and Lehmann and Ryan in 1956 related suxamethonium apnoea to abnormalities of the enzyme.

Plasma cholinesterase is determined genetically mainly by two allelomorphic genes on an autosomal chromosome (not sex-linked). There are four genes:

- Normal or Usual: N or E_1^u
- Dibucaine-resistant or Atypical: D or E_1^a
- Fluoride-resistant: F or E_1^f
- Silent: S or E_1^s

A further gene on another chromosome, the C5 variant, results in an increased level of plasma cholinesterase activity. Table 8.2 shows these genetic variations.

The scoline number is increasingly used as a guide to the abnormality of plasma cholinesterase as it reflects the metabolism of suxamethonium most accurately. A high number indicates a normal response to suxamethonium.

The dibucaine number is the % inhibition by 10^{-5} M dibucaine (1×10^{-5} mol/l). The D gene produces cholinesterase resistant to inhibition.

The fluoride number is the % inhibition by 5×10^{-5} M fluoride (5×10^{-5} mol/l).

The genes display individual variation, leading to a range of values in the tests. The N gene is dominant in heterozygotes.

Mendelian inheritance determines the genotype of a child. Each allele of an ovum can combine with each one of a sperm in this manner: $N_1N_1 + N_2N_2$ produce $N_1N_2 + N_1N_2 + N_2N_1 + N_2N_1$. Hence *two heterozygotes will result in one normal and one abnormal homozygotes and two heterozygotes:* $N_1D_1 + N_2D_2 = N_1N_2 + D_1D_2 + N_1D_2 + N_2D_1$. By the same rearrangement it will be seen that a normal homozygous (NN) and a heterozygous (ND) mating will produce equal numbers of normal homozygous and heterozygous offspring. Table 8:3 correlates the genotypic variations of plasma cholinesterase with the phenotypic expression (duration of apnoea) and the frequency with which this has been reported.

Table 8.2 Genetic variants of plasma, cholinesterase. (The numbers in brackets are averages, as an aid to memory.)

Genotype	Activity, units/l	Suxamethonium sensitivity	Dibucaine number	Fluoride number	Scoline number	Incidence
NN	677–1560	Normal	77–83 (80)	56–68 (60)	88–95 (90)	96%
ND	474–1110	Some increase	48–69 (60)	44–54 (50)	56–77 (65)	4%
DD	166–757	Very high	8–28 (20)	10–28 (20)	4–25 (15)	1:3000
NF	611–1150	Slight increase	70–83 (75)	48–54 (50)	84–91 (90)	1:200
NS	385–870	Slight increase	77–83 (80)	56–68 (60)	86–93 (90)	1:200
DF	475–648	Increased	45–59 (50)	28–39 (35)	54–60 (55)	1:20 000
DS	96–489	Very high	8–28 (20)	10–28 (20)	4–28 (15)	1:30 000
FF	0	Very high	64–69 (67)	34–43 (40)	0	1:150 000
FS	351–509	Very high	64–69 (67)	34–43 (40)	80–81 (80)	1:100 000
SS	0–48	Very high	0	0	0	1:10 000

Table 8.3   Apnoea with abnormal plasma cholinesterase

% of reports	Genotype	Duration (minutes)
71.0	DD	12–240
11.0	ND	7–60
8.0	DS	45–210
2.5	NS	85–120
2.5	DF	20–60
2.0	SS	70–330
1.5	NF	10–20
0.5	FS	30

In addition to inherited variations, plasma cholinesterase activity may be influenced by *physiological, acquired or iatrogenic factors* (see Table 8.4). An important clinical example is patients with **burns**. The rate and magnitude of fall of plasma cholinesterase is related to the severity of the burn. Activity is depressed by the 6th day, and may fall by 80%. It remains low for months in severe cases despite healing.

Cholinesterase poisoning

1. Phosphonium insecticides are used as agricultural pesticides. They are readily absorbed by the lungs, skin and conjunctivae, binding irreversibly to plasma cholinesterase. Regeneration of the enzyme has been attempted with

Table 8.4   Variations in plasma cholinesterase levels (Whittaker 1981)

	Decreased activity	Increased activity
Inherited	Abnormal variants	Very rare variants (C5)
Physiological	2–3 days postpartum	6/12 to 5 years
	Neonates	
Acquired	Liver disease (inflammatory, metastases)	Obesity
	Myocardial infarction	Nodular goitre
	Collagen diseases	Thyrotoxicosis
	Myxoedema	Nephrosis
	Malignancy	Anxiety
	Cachexia	Alcoholism
	Chronic anaemia	Psoriasis
	Uraemia	Asthma
	Burns (see text)	Hypertension
Iatrogenic	Organophosphate insecticides	
	Ecothiopate	
	Neostigmine	
	Metoclopramide	
	MAO inhibitors	
	Pancuronium	
	Cyclophosphamide	
	Contraceptive pills	
	Cytotoxics	
	X-ray therapy.	

aldoximes (2-PAM, DAM). The emphasis of treatment remains supportive, i.e. counteracting the cerebral and neuromuscular blocking effects.

2. Ecothiopate (Phospholine) eyedrops used in glaucoma also lower plasma cholinesterase level.

REVERSIBLE ANTICHOLINESTERASES

Neostigmine (Prostigmine), t½β 30–130 min, or **pyridostigmine** (Mestinon) t½β 101–125 min, reduce the intensity of non-depolarizing block by inhibiting acetylcholinesterase.

Neostigmine attaches to ACh-esterase to form a Michaelis–Menten complex similar to that formed by ACh, but hydrolysed far less quickly (t½ 0.5 h). Part is thus metabolized (30%), the remainder being excreted unchanged in the urine. Neostigmine has a quaternary nitrogen, producing some direct cholinergic action, and making it highly polar so that it cannot cross the blood–brain barrier (in contrast to physostigmine).

Pyridostigmine in a dose of 10 mg (with atropine 1 mg) has been proposed as an alternative to neostigmine on the basis of reports that it causes less bradycardia and secretions, but its onset is slower.

Edrophonium has a quaternary nitrogen group and can increase ACh release, producing fasciculations. Higher doses (0.5–1.0 mg/kg) are necessary as it has a shorter half-life.

Physostigmine (Eserine) is a non-polar anticholinesterase and crosses the blood–brain barrier. It has been used to antagonize the delirium due to overdosage with scopolamine.

Table 8.5 outlines the equivalent doses, onset and elimination of neostigmine, pyridostigmine and edrophonium.

Tetrahydroaminacrine (THA) inhibits plasma cholinesterase more than acetylcholinesterase and prolongs the action of suxamethonium. It is also a non-specific stimulator of the CNS. *Hexafluorenium* also prolongs the effect of suxamethonium.

4 Amino-pyridine (4 A-P)

4 A-P blocks the exit of K^+ and prolongs the action potential. It enhances the entry of Ca^{2+} and hence the release of ACh. It is not an anticholinesterase. It antagonises the block caused by the mycin antibiotics, and has been used

Table 8.5 Equivalent doses, onset and elimination. (Elimination is prolonged in impaired renal function.)

Drug	Dose, mg/kg	Onset, minutes	t½ elimination, minutes
Neostigmine (Prostigmine)	0.05	3.5	80 ± 50
Pyridostigmine (Mestinon)	0.20	8.0	113 ± 12
Edrophonium (Tensilon)	0.50	2.0	35 ± 10

in the myasthenic syndrome of Eaton–Lambert (associated with malignant disease, especially of the lung). 4 A-P also reverses the block produced by botulinus toxin experimentally, a form of 'open-channel' block affecting the nerve ending. Dosage is 0.6 mg/kg; Vd, 2.6 ± 1.0 l/kg; $t\frac{1}{2}\beta$, 3.5 ± 1.0 h. It is excreted 98% unchanged by the kidney. Effective doses cause unacceptable CNS stimulation. It enhances the effectiveness of anticholinesterases: 0.3 mg/kg, and reduces the requirement of neostigmine from 0.05 to 0.01 mg/kg.

Germine monoacetate has actions similar to 4 A-P.

THE IDEAL NEUROMUSCULAR BLOCKING DRUG

1. Non-depolarizing action
2. Rapid onset (one circulation time)
3. Short duration (suitable for infusion) or duration about 0.5 h
4. Rapid metabolism to inactive products
5. Antagonized by anticholinesterase
6. Actions confined to NMJ
7. No significant transfer across placenta or blood–brain barrier
8. No local or systemic side-effects (e.g. histamine release)
9. Compatibility with other drugs and injections
10. Long shelf-life without special storage (e.g. refrigeration)
11. Not expensive: synthesis not too complex
12. Sterilizable.

NEUROMUSCULAR BLOCK AND MUSCLE RELAXANTS

History

1857 Claude Bernard: curare acts on the NMJ
1935 King: curare isolated in pure form
1944 Griffith and McIntyre: use in anaesthetics
1946 Bovet: first synthetic analogue (gallamine)
1951 Depolarizing block (suxamethonium) used clinically.

Chemistry

Molecules with two quaternary nitrogen atoms separated by 1.2–1.5 nm (12–15 Angstrom units) mimic or block the effects of ACh at the NMJ. They may also be atropine-like, have local anaesthetic properties and be anticholinesterases. The quaternary nitrogen is related to the ammonium ion, NH_4^+, with the hydrogens replaced with methyl groups: $N(CH_3)_4^+$.

Non-depolarizing block is associated with:

1. high ionization (polarity)
2. a positively-charged (cationic) centre

3. a molecular configuration which allows the cationic centre to approach the receptor closely.

Types of neuromuscular block

1. Non-depolarizing (NDB)
2. Depolarizing (DB)
3. Phase II (when DB is prolonged)
4. Open-channel
5. Closed-channel
6. Deficiency.

Non-depolarizing block

a. If incomplete, increased ACh (by an anticholinesterase) antagonizes the block: the block is competitive.
b. Recovery occurs when the blocker is removed.
c. Repetitive stimuli cause **fade** due to ACh depletion.
d. Muscle groups vary in sensitivity.
e. Effects of two NDBs are additive (or supra-additive if one has prejunctional effects also).
f. A positive electrode hyperpolarizes the membrane, increasing block. A negative one opposes it.
g. A threshold dose is necessary to initiate block as 80% of receptors have to be blocked to reduce transmission (the margin of safety: see Table 8.1). Hence recovery occurs before the drug is fully eliminated.
h. Repeated stimulation followed by a pause then a single stimulus produces **posttetanic facilitation** – a supranormal twitch.
i. Hypothermia decreases the intensity of NDB, probably by slowing the rate of hydrolysis of ACh. The duration of atracurium is increased.
j. Respiratory alkalosis reduces the block produced by atracurium, vecuronium or tubocurarine but does not affect that of pancuronium or alcuronium.
k. Acidosis increases the block, except for alcuronium (no effect).
l. Volatile anaesthetics enhance block by decreasing the activity of moto-neurones, and in higher concentration depressing the skeletal muscles.
m. A fall of K^+ hyperpolarizes the postjunctional membrane and increases NDB. A rise has the opposite effect.
n. The **change in end-plate potential** (– 90 mv) decreases until the EPP fails to reach threshold (about – 70 mv), preventing propagation to the muscle fibre (the **action potential**). (See Fig. 8.5.)
o. **Offset of block** is hastened by redistribution to **acceptor sites:** pharmacodynamically inactive receptors which bind NDBs. They are mucopolysaccharides, mainly in lungs, liver, muscle and cartilage.

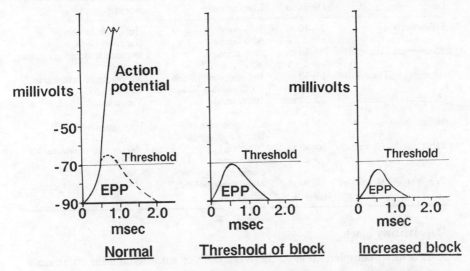

Fig. 8.5 Changes in end-plate potential (EPP). Most of the end-plate potential is obscured by the muscle action potential until block occurs. Block is **all-or-none** for each junction: the gradual fall in power is due to increasing numbers of blocked junctions. This implies a variable susceptibility to non-depolarizing block (NDB) and probably variations in perfusion and drug access.

Prolonged dosage saturates them, after which the offset of action of the NDBs is much slower, being dependent on elimination: this may be seen when paralysis is prolonged for many hours in the intensive care unit.

p. In the elderly the number of receptors falls, with increased sensitivity to NDBs. The number of glomeruli falls, with slower renal excretion. Extracellular water also falls, with a lower Vd. Hence dosage requirement decreases, and duration is increased.

NON-DEPOLARIZING NEUROMUSCULAR BLOCKERS

In clinical practice the choice of non-depolarizing blocker depends on duration of action, side-effects and routes of elimination of the drugs (see Table 8.6). The introduction of drugs which undergo extensive metabolism has made some earlier ones obsolescent. The introduction of monitoring techniques has increased the versatility of the intermediate duration agents vecuronium and atracurium.

Pipecuronium and doxacuronium are very long-acting and excreted unchanged: their probable role is uncertain.

Table 8.6 Non-depolarizing blockers Note: In clinical use, duration increases with a high initial dose and volatile anaesthetic supplements: enflurane reduces the dose requirement of d-tubocurarine by about 66%. Isoflurane and halothane are less effective.

Drug	Duration	Elimination	Side-effects
d-Tubocurarine	30–40 m t½β 2 ± 1 h	70% renal 30% biliary	Histamine release Ganglion block
Alcuronium (Alloferin)	30–40 m t½β 2 ± 1 h	70% renal 30% biliary	Immune response reported
Atracurium (Tracrium)	15–30 m t½β 20 m	Hoffman degradation, cholinesterase hydrolysis	No vagolysis: bradycardia may occur
Gallamine (Flaxedil)	20–30 m t½β 2.5 h	100% renal	Tachycardia
Mivacurium	15–20 m	Cholinesterase and biliary hydrolysis.	No vagolysis
Pancuronium (Pavulon)	30–40 m t½β 2 h	70% renal 30% biliary (some hydroxylated)	Noradrenaline release: tachycardia
Vecuronium (Norcuron)	15–30 m t½β 1 h	Mainly metabolized: biliary	No vagolysis: bradycardia

Depolarizing block

a. It is often complete, due to the large dose of suxamethonium commonly used affecting all receptors.
b. There is no antagonist.
c. If incomplete, a twitch response is possible, and a tetanus will be sustained (that is, there is no fade).
d. Non-depolarizing drugs given as a pre-dose lessen the intensity of the response: a larger dose of suxamethonium is necessary.
e. Block is prolonged with added cholinergic drugs.
f. Some muscles e.g. extraocular ones respond with a 'contracture' instead of a contraction and relaxation. This increases intraocular pressure for some minutes.

This type of block is seen with suxamethonium, but may occur with drugs which delay the hydrolysis of ACh (overdose of neostigmine), or prolonged stimulation with a negative electrode (prolonged depolarization).

Prolonged block results in **desensitization** of the membrane adjacent to the NMJ: even when an end-plate potential can be evoked, it is not conducted to the muscle. The longer the period of stimulation, the slower the recovery from the desensitization.

Phase II block

This appears with repeated doses of depolarizing blocker, features follow:

1. If a tetanus can be produced, fade occurs: the train-of-four ratio decreases.
2. Recovery is slower.
3. Neostigmine decreases the intensity of block. If neostigmine is given before all the suxamethonium has been hydrolysed, it will prolong the life of

the drug by slowing its further hydrolysis, and enhance the development of phase II block. Hence neostigmine should not be used until phase II block is confirmed by a fade in response to a tetanus.

Open-channel block

Some drugs can enter and block open ion channels: barbiturates, verapamil, some antibiotics, local anaesthetics. Block is non-competitive, and enhanced by ACh (which opens the channels: neostigmine may thus enhance this block).

Closed-channel block

Ion channels can be blocked at their entrance by some antibiotics, quinidine, naloxone, naltrexone and tricyclic antidepressants.

Deficiency block

The lessening release of ACh with a tetanus leads to increased non-depolarizing (ND) block. Any reduction in motor neurone discharge (deep anaesthesia) or nerve conduction (spinal or conduction block with local anaesthetics) will also lead to lowered ACh release.

Botulinus toxin, hypocalcaemia or increased magnesium concentration impair the release of ACh.

SUXAMETHONIUM: ACTIONS OTHER THAN MUSCLE RELAXATION

1. Fasciculations

These are fibrillary tremors of skeletal muscles, probably due to stimulation of the motor nerve ending by suxamethonium. Antidromic impulses produce an axon reflex so that groups of muscle fibres become stimulated. These are apparently not related to muscle pains. Reduced by prior partial non-depolarizing block or a small dose of suxamethonium itself.

2. Muscle pains

Occur frequently, especially if early ambulation is allowed (up to 66%). Less common in children, more common in females. Chest wall pain is common, being likened to the discomfort expected after cardiac compression via the chest wall: the patient may wrongly suspect that a circulatory arrest has occurred. Incidence greatly decreased by a previous small dose of NDB.

3. Bradycardia

Initially reported after repeated doses in children, but also seen in adults. Vagotonic in origin and prevented by atropine.

4. Potassium release

Plasma potassium rises slightly in normal patients, but to a hazardous level in **burns** (especially if these are deep) from the 6th day (corresponding to the fall in plasma cholinesterase), and from the week following **spinal cord transection.** Thought to be due to increased sensitivity of postjunctional receptors: the rise in potassium may cause cardiac arrest in diastole.

5. Raised intraocular pressure

This may be due to prolonged contraction (contracture) of extraocular muscles, and may cause vitreous loss if the eye is open.

6. Raised intra-abdominal pressure

This may cause regurgitation of gastric content in a non-fasted patient. It may be reduced by pretreating with 10% of the intubating dose of a NDB, given 2–3 min before suxamethonium. The dose of suxamethonium should then be increased by 50%.

7. Masseter spasm

This was thought to be an early sign of the risk of malignant hyperthermia, but in fact occurs commonly. It may be a problem in myotonia congenita by reducing access for laryngoscopy.

METABOLISM OF SUXAMETHONIUM

About 90% of the dose injected is destroyed before it reaches the NMJ. If plasma cholinesterase is abnormal or absent, about 10% of the usual dose produces clinical paralysis, with duration similar to the non-depolarizers.

Suxamethonium is hydrolysed in two steps. Succinylmonocholine (plus choline) occurs first, and this metabolite has up to 10% of the blocking activity of the parent. Although succinylmonocholine is hydrolysed more slowly than succinyldicholine (suxamethonium), it is unlikely to cause prolonged paralysis unless very large doses of suxamethonium have been given. The kidney excretes 14%, and the remainder is hydrolysed to succinic acid and choline.

With *abnormal plasma cholinesterase*, some undergoes alkaline hydrolysis in the blood (pH 7.4) but it is very variable, so that duration of paralysis is unpredictable (see Table 8.3). Alkaline hydrolysis removes about 5% per hour, and renal excretion occurs with a $t_{1/2}\beta$ of about 1 h.

Note: Suxamethonium undergoes spontaneous hydrolysis in solution in the presence of heat and light. At room temperature (20°C) it loses 5% of its potency in 3 months, and 20% in 12 months: supplies should be kept refrigerated.

FURTHER READING

Whittaker M 1981 In: Ellis F R (ed.) Inherited disease and anesthesia, Excerpta Medica. Elsevier, Amsterdam, ch 4, p 105–126

9. Local anaesthetics

DESIRABLE PROPERTIES

Pharmacodynamic:

a. Reversible depression of conduction
b. Sensory > motor depression
c. Specific action confined to nerve tissue
d. Freedom from cellular injury, especially neural and hepatic.

Pharmacokinetic:

a. Effective topically on mucosae
b. Rapid onset of action without initial pain
c. Adequate duration for surgery or long-term analgesia
d. Is metabolized rather than requiring renal excretion.

Toxicity:

Low systemic toxicity if injected into the circulation inadvertently.

Physical properties:

a. Water-soluble
b. Sterilizable by heat
c. Stable when exposed to light, air or pH changes
d. Compatible with vasoconstrictor solutions; adrenaline, felypressin.

TYPES OF AGENTS

Esters

Formed by condensation of an organic acid and aminoalcohol.

Cocaine: benzoic acid and ecgonine (the base is closely related to tropine, the base of atropine).
Procaine: para-aminobenzoic acid and diethyl aminoethanol.

Nesacaine is 2-chloroprocaine: it undergoes hydrolysis faster than any other local anaesthetic (LA).

Amethocaine (Decicaine, Anethaine, Pontocaine) is used as a surface anaesthetic.

Other esters are obsolete.

Aminoamides

Lignocaine (Xylocaine, Lidocaine)   Prilocaine (Citanest)
Bupivacaine (Marcain)   Mepivacaine (Carbocaine)
Etidocaine (Duranest)   Ropivacaine
Cinchocaine (Nupercaine, Percaine, Dibucaine)

Note: Local anaesthetic properties are common among drugs, especially antihistamines, beta-adrenoreceptor blockers and biological toxins.

PHARMACODYNAMICS

The action of the local anaesthetics on nerve cells follows entry into the cell (see below in Pharmacokinetic section). The ionized base inhibits the 'm' gate of the ion channel, preventing the entry of Na^+ and consequent depolarization. The membrane is said to be 'stabilized'. Table 9.1 gives specific pharmacodynamic information regarding the commonly used local anaesthetics.

PHARMACOKINETICS

Pharmacokinetic characteristics of various local anaesthetics are given in Table 9.2.

Physical characteristics

1. Lipid solubility

This determines the rate of entry into nerve tissue and affects the duration of action. It falls in the order: etidocaine > bupivacaine > lignocaine > prilocaine.

Table 9.1 Pharmacodynamics of local anaesthetics

	% Equipotent concentration	Dose mg/kg	Toxic level, µg/ml
Lignocaine	1.00	5 (7 with adrenaline)	6–8
Bupivacaine	0.25	2	2
Etidocaine	0.50	5	2
Prilocaine	1.00	6 (8 with adrenaline)	7
Procaine	1.50	5 (7 with adrenaline)	7–10

Table 9.2   Pharmacokinetic data

	pK_a	% Plasma protein binding (PPB)	Plasma $t_{\frac{1}{2}\beta}$ (hours)	Onset	Duration (hours)	% Hepatic extraction
Lignocaine	7.7	70	2.6	Fast	1–2	68
Bupivacaine	8.1	96	2.4	Medium	2–6	37
Etidocaine	7.7	94	2.4	Fast	2–6	73
Procaine	8.9	3		Medium	0.5–0.75	
Cocaine	8.6				Topical	
Prilocaine	7.7	55	1.5	Fast	1–2	
Mepivacaine	7.6	75	2.0	Slow	1.5–3.0	
Ropivacaine	8.1			Medium	4–6	
Cinchocaine	8.5			Slow	2–3	

Entry to the nerve cell and subsequent blocking is related to the ratio of ionized/un-ionized drug (which is unity at the pK_a). Hence as the value of the pK_a approaches the pH of extracellular fluid the onset becomes faster due to an increased lipid-soluble fraction.

Local anaesthetics are mainly *bases*. Their chloride salts are water-soluble, and are highly ionized in solution. *Their pK_as are higher than the pH of tissue fluid:* the higher the pK_a the less free base is available to enter lipid membranes. On entry, the cellular pH is lower than that of extracellular fluid and ionization increases further.

A salt of the LA base with a weak acid (carbonic) will hydrolyze more readily in extracellular fluid than one with a mineral acid (hydrochloric). The enhanced release of free base will increase the rate of onset: with carbonated lignocaine onset occurs in one-quarter of the time taken by the chloride, but the carbonate is less stable chemically, limiting its usefulness.

2. Concentration of the solution

A stronger solution increases the rate of onset and duration, but not in proportion. Because the total dose is limited by toxicity, smaller volumes only can be used with concentrated solutions.

3. Additives

Adrenaline: this decreases tissue perfusion and increases the rate of onset and duration of action. This effect is less marked with the very lipid-soluble drugs (bupivacaine) whose offset is determined by the rate of release from neural tissue. *Procaine* is a vasodilator, and its action is markedly increased by adrenaline. *Ropivacaine* is a vasoconstrictor and this may obviate the need for adrenaline, thus increasing its compatibility with halogenated anaesthetics.

Adrenaline is a weak local anaesthetic, intensifying motor block particularly. This effect is seen after subarachnoid or epidural injection.

4. Temperature

A warmed solution acts faster.

Site of application

1. Nerve diameter and myelination

B-fibres (preganglionic sympathetics) are most susceptible. A-fibres (motor, sensory) are next, and C-fibres (subserving deep pain) are most resistant. In a mixed nerve the outermost fibres, irrespective of their size, are likely to be affected first by LA injected nearby.

2. Local factors

Vascularity Absorption from the site of injection decreases in this order: intercostal block > tracheal spray > plexus anaesthesia > epidural block > local infiltration.

Skin application The penetration of local anaesthetics is too limited to produce anaesthesia unless they are especially prepared. EMLA (Eutectic Mixture of Local Anaesthetics – lignocaine and prilocaine bases: the eutectic mixture remains liquid at room temperature) is the only available example. EMLA takes about an hour to penetrate sufficiently, depending on the thickness of the stratum corneum, but lasts for a further hour or more. Amethocaine has since been shown to work similarly.

Note: Transdermal cream is very concentrated, and toxic levels are readily exceeded if the cream is accidentally swallowed (e.g. small children).

Mucosal application A pK_a closer to neutrality favours absorption: lignocaine (pK_a 7.7) is effective, but procaine (pK_a 8.9) is not.

Factors related to the patient

1. Alpha-1-acid glycoprotein (AAG)

AAG is mainly responsible for protein binding of LA. Its level falls during *pregnancy*. The resultant increase in the 'free fraction' increases the risk of toxicity (and, for the same reason, the effectiveness of the LAs). The *AAG level rises in renal failure*, reducing the free fraction, and the associated renal metabolic acidosis increases the ionization of the base: these two factors markedly shorten the duration of action of LA.

2. Age

The t½β for plasma elimination is 2–3 times longer in the neonate. For lignocaine it is 4 h, for mepivacaine 10 h. Volume of distribution falls, and plasma t½β increases by 70% in old age.

3. Systemic disease

Normal patients have a high liver blood flow (25% of cardiac output) and high liver extraction and metabolism. Hence elimination will be slower in liver disease or heart failure (see Table 9.3) or with drugs that reduce liver blood flow: metoprolol or propranolol reduce clearance by 30%; general anaesthesia (with halothane, for example) also reduces clearance by up to 30%.

Metabolism

Procaine, an ester, is hydrolysed by plasma cholinesterase into inert metabolites.

The aminoamides are metabolized by liver enzymes.

Lignocaine has a high hepatic extraction: its t½β is 2.6 h. It is dealkylated and hydrolysed to a xylidine derivative which is excreted by the kidney. A minor intermediate, glycine-xylidide, has a long t½β and is also an LA.

Bupivacaine has a lower hepatic clearance: 3 mlkg^{-1}min^{-1}, and is metabolized slowly to inert compounds.

Ropivacaine clearance is about 6 mlkg^{-1}min^{-1}, a factor which, it is suggested, increases its margin of safety.

Prilocaine is rapidly broken down, mainly in the liver but also by the kidneys and lungs. O-toluidine which is formed causes methaemoglobin-aemia.

Mepivacaine, in patients aged more than a few weeks, is rapidly broken down to inert metabolites in the liver. The **neonate has immature liver enzyme development** and the t½β is **10 h**: the persisting drug causes detectable behavioural disturbances.

TOXICITY

1. *Local injury* may occur mechanically from direct needle trauma to the nerve, or from disruption and pressure ischaemia from injecting into the inelastic nerve-sheath. Chemical injury is very rare with currently available drugs; additives such as metabisulphite (an antioxidant) have been implicated.

Table 9.3 Lignocaine pharmacokinetics in disease

	Plasma t½β (hours)	Volume of distribution (l/kg)	Clearance (mlkg^{-1}min^{-1})
Normal	1.6	1.32	10.0
Heart failure	1.9	0.88	6.3
Liver diseae	4.9	2.31	6.0
Renal disease	1.3	1.2	13.7

2. *Generalized toxicity* is related to blood level and is dependent on:

1. total dosage
2. rate of absorption into the circulation (decreased by adrenaline)
3. rate of elimination.

Inadvertent intravenous injection is the commonest cause of generalized toxicity. Effects may follow a dose below the recommended maximum because there is insufficient time for the drug to become bound to plasma protein (as occurs during slow absorption) and the peak free-fraction is correspondingly higher. This is especially important with **bupivacaine** which is highly bound and also cardiotoxic.

The increased cardiotoxicity of bupivacaine is related to its effects on sodium channels: it is fast-in and slow-out, whereas lignocaine is fast-in and fast-out. **Relative cardiotoxicity of bupivacaine:lignocaine is 16:1.**

3. *Safety ratios of blood levels causing circulatory depression: CNS toxicity are lignocaine 7:1, bupivacaine 4:1.*

4. *Prilocaine and methaemoglobinaemia:* 0.3 mg/kg prilocaine produces 1 g of methaemoglobin; 400 mg of prilocaine in a 70 kg patient (600 mg if adrenaline is added) may produce clinical cyanosis after some delay. This will resolve spontaneously in 12 h, or may be treated with methylene blue 1 mg/kg, or ascorbic acid.

5. *Toxic effects: CNS and CVS*
For lignocaine:
   4 µg/ml – light-headedness, tinnitus, circumoral numbness
   6 µg/ml – visual disturbance
   8 µg/ml – muscle twitching
   10 µg/ml – convulsions
   12 µg/ml – unconsciousness
   20 µg/ml – respiratory arrest
   24 µg/ml – circulatory depression.

Lignocaine is a class 1B antiarrhythmic (see Chapter 11). It stabilizes excitable membranes, and acts by slowing the rate of depolarization and shortening the action potential in ischaemic myocardium.

Prophylaxis against CNS toxicity can be achieved with diazepam 0.1 mg/kg. Diazepam is highly plasma protein-bound, and this would tend to increase the toxicity of bupivacaine and etidocaine which are also highly bound (95%) by displacing them and thus increasing the free fraction.

Treatment of toxicity

This includes respiratory support with oxygen and administration of an anticonvulsant. Thiopentone 1–3 mg/kg given slowly is very effective, or diazepam 0.1 mg/kg. A neuromuscular blocker may be necessary to control violent movements. Circulatory depression with bupivacaine is very resistant to treatment: re-entrant arrhythmias may occur. Bretylium tosylate (Bretylate) is a specific antidote, raising the threshold for ventricular fibrillation (see Chapter 11).

10. Vasoactive drugs

THE CATECHOLAMINES

Adrenal medullary amines

Adrenaline – main circulating hormone in adults.

Noradrenaline – minor circulating hormone except in the fetus; transmitter at postganglionic sympathetic endings.

Dopamine – precursor to noradrenaline. Inotropic to heart and vasodilates renal vessels at low concentration. Transmitter in CNS in thalamus, hypothalamus and basal ganglia.

Distribution

Adrenal medulla

Adrenaline is stored in some cells, and released by insulin. Noradrenaline (NA) is stored in other cells and is depleted by reserpine or guanethidine. Nerve stimuli release varying proportions of amines: noradrenaline predominates in fetal life but constitutes 20% in adults.

Other sites

Postganglionic sympathetic nerves are noradrenergic except sweat glands and pilomotor muscles which are cholinergic. Some sympathetic postganglionic nerves release ACh which then releases noradrenaline from chromaffin cells found near blood vessels in skin, lungs, bladder, heart, uterus and skeletal muscle.

Adrenergic receptors

Alpha-receptors and beta-receptors

$Alpha_1$ *stimulate* vascular smooth muscle (except skeletal muscle vessels), the radial muscle of the pupil (mydriasis) and smooth muscle in the splenic capsule, erector pilae (gooseflesh), biliary tract and vas deferens. They *inhibit* intestinal smooth muscle except sphincters.

119

Typical *alpha₁ agonists* are *methoxamine and phenylephrine. Antagonists* include *phenoxybenzamine* (Dibenyline, very long-acting) and *prazosin* (Minipress).

Alpha₂ are found presynaptically on adrenergic nerve endings (where they are inhibitory to NA release), on platelets (increasing aggregation) and in the CNS.

Clonidine (Catapres) and *dexmedetomidine* are agonists, and *yohimbine* an antagonist.

Antagonists for alpha₁ and alpha₂ are common: *phentolamine* (Rogitine, short-acting, competitive), *ergotamine, tolazoline* (Priscol), the *phenothiazines* and *butyrophenones.*

Beta₁ are found in the heart (increased rate and force of contraction) and smooth muscle of the gut (decreased motility).

Noradrenaline and *dobutamine* (Dobutrex) are beta₁ agonists.

Beta₂ are predominantly inhibitory: bronchodilation, vasodilation in skeletal muscle vessels, uterine relaxation, decreased motility of gut. They subserve glycogenolysis and (together with alpha receptors) gluconeogenesis.

Salbutamol (Ventolin), *terbutaline* (Bricanyl), *orciprenaline* (Alupent) and *fenoterol* (Berotec) are *agonists* and are used mainly in bronchial asthma.

Isoprenaline was the first beta agonist described but its cardiac (beta₁) effects limited its use.

Table 10.1 lists the commonly used beta-receptor antagonists, their relative affinity to receptor subtypes and pharmacokinetics. Table 10.2 gives a full list of alpha- and beta-receptor agonists.

Alpha- and beta-receptors are blocked by *labetalol* (Trandate) which has a t½β of 4 h. It has been reported as causing profound hypotension during halothane anaesthesia. The beta blockade is 7 times the intensity of the alpha blockade.

In summary, the alpha actions are stimulatory except for the effects on the gut, and the beta actions are inhibitory except for the effect on the heart.

Table 10.1 Beta-adrenoreceptor blockers

Drug	Beta₁	Beta₂	Partial agonist	Bioavailability	t½β
Alprenolol (Aptin)	+	+	+ +	Low	2–3 h
Atenolol (Tenormin)	+	0	0	Moderate	6–9 h
Metoprolol (Betaloc)	+	0	0	Moderate	3–4 h
Oxprenolol (Trasicor)	+	+	+ +	Moderate	2 h
Pindolol (Visken)	+	+	+ + +	High	3–4 h
Propranolol (Inderal)	+	+	0	Moderate	4–6 h
Timolol (Timoptol)	+	+	0	High	4–5 h
Esmolol (Brevibloc)	+	0	+	i.v.	9 min

Table 10.2 Adrenergic drugs

Drug	Alpha$_1$	Alpha$_2$	Beta$_1$	Beta$_2$	Comments
Adrenaline	+ +	+ +	+ +	+ +	
Noradrenaline	+ +	+ +	+	+	0.5–1.5 µgkg^{-1}min^{-1}
Isoprenaline	+		+ +	+ +	
Dopamine	+ +		+ + +	+	1–2 µgkg^{-1}min^{-1} increases renal blood flow direct tubular diuretic effect 2–10 µgkg^{-1}min^{-1} increases cardiac output
Dobutamine	+ (> 10 µgkg^{-1} min^{-1})		+ +	+ +	Short t½β Dopaminergic on renal blood flow Rate 2.5–10 µgkg^{-1}min^{-1}
Dopexamine				+ +	Dopaminergic
Phenylephrine	+				
Methoxamine	+				
Ephedrine	+	+	+	+	Indirect action
Clonidine		+			See p. 126
Metaraminol	+ +	+			Mainly indirect
Salbutamol				+ +	Bronchodilator Uterine relaxation
Terbutaline				+ +	Bronchodilator
Fenoterol				+ +	Bronchodilator

Dopaminergic receptors

- DA$_1$ relax renal vessels and gut smooth muscle.
- DA$_2$ mediate presynaptic inhibition of release of dopamine and NA.
- CNS effects: DA$_1$ affect extrapyramidal activity. DA$_2$ affect the release of endorphins and ACh, and inhibit pituitary hormone release.

Glucagon and angiotensin II

Glucagon, a polypeptide from the alpha pancreatic cells, is an inotrope acting by adenylate cyclase. It also causes hyperglycaemia and hyperkalaemia.

Angiotensin II, an octapeptide, is derived from angiotensin I by the action of plasma peptidase. Captopril (Capoten) and enalapril (Renitec) inhibit this conversion. Angiotensin I is derived from an alpha$_2$ globulin, angiotensinogen, by the action of renin which is released from the renal cortex. Angiotensin II is a potent vasoconstrictor, increasing peripheral resistance and diastolic pressure, but reducing splanchnic blood flow.

Hazards

1. Most antagonists affect both beta$_1$ and beta$_2$ receptors, precluding their use in hypertensive patients who also have asthma. Atenolol and metoprolol (see Table 10.1) are cardiospecific, reducing this hazard.

2. Patients with compensated cardiac failure can be precipitated into acute cardiac failure by beta blockade.

3. The combinations of beta-blocking and calcium ion channel-blocking drugs can readily lead to bradycardia and a profound fall in cardiac output especially during anaesthesia.

Note: Adrenergic blocking drugs frequently have **partial agonist activity** *(intrinsic sympathomimetic activity or ISA)* and their action on various receptors is often concentration-dependent, as is also seen with the agonists (as the infusion rate increases, dopamine initially causes renal vasodilation, then cardiac inotropy, and then profound vasoconstriction including the renal vessels).

Release of noradrenaline (See Fig. 10.1)

Mediated by cyclic AMP and Ca^{2+} entry into the nerve ending. Modified predominantly by two prejunctional receptors: $alpha_2$ and $beta_2$.

Alpha$_2$ receptors are acted on by noradrenaline (NA) in the synaptic cleft, reducing the amount of Ca^{2+} available for excitation–secretion coupling and limiting NA release: an example of negative feedback. Alpha antagonists (phentolamine) decrease this action.

Beta$_2$ receptors are stimulated by circulating adrenaline. They increase the synthesis of cyclic AMP and NA release: positive feedback. They are inhibited by beta-antagonists (propranolol), and enhanced by beta-agonists (salbutamol).

Other prejunctional receptors may increase (+) or decrease (–) stimulation-induced NA release: prostaglandin E_1 and E_2 (–), enkephalin

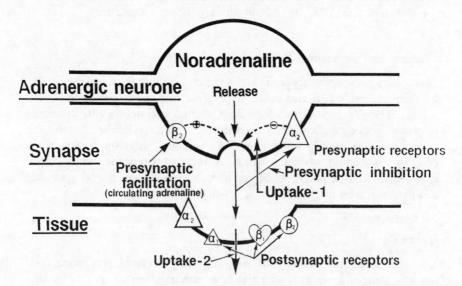

Fig. 10.1 The adrenergic synapse. See text for explanation.

opiate receptors (–), dopamine (–), muscarinic ACh (–), nicotinic ACh (+), adenosine (–), angiotensin II (+).

Re-uptake of noradrenaline (See Fig. 10.1)

Most of the released NA is rapidly taken up by the adrenergic neurone. Re-uptake is inhibited by cocaine, tricyclic antidepressants, guanethidine and reserpine: an enhanced initial response may thus occur due to the accumulated NA. A decreased response then follows as NA becomes depleted. This will reduce the effect of *indirectly-acting adrenergic drugs* (those which act by NA release: ephedrine, metaraminol (Aramine), tyramine), but directly-acting drugs (methoxamine, adrenaline) are unaffected.

Metabolism of adrenaline and noradrenaline

NA which is not taken up by the adrenergic ending (*uptake 1*) undergoes metabolism by *catechol-O-methyl transferase (COMT)* and *monoamine oxidase (MAO)*, two enzymes widely available in the tissues. Tissue absorption is termed *uptake 2*. Adrenaline undergoes the same fate.

COMT replaces the 3-OH group on the catechol molecule with a CH_3O group, initiating the process which alters the molecule to 3-methoxy-4-hydroxy-mandelic acid (VMA).

MAO in the adrenergic ending contributes to the physiological balance of free and granular NA. MAO is widely distributed. The 'A' type enzyme acts mainly on polar aromatic amines (serotonin, NA), the 'B' type on non-polar aromatic amines (phenylethylamine, benzylamine). Irreversible inhibitors are associated with dietary reactions (see Chapter 14) and MAO-A inhibitors are being developed as they avoid this risk, and show promise of being faster-acting. A reversible MAO-B inhibitor (selegiline, or Deprenyl) is also free of dietary reactions and allows a 25% reduction of the dose of levodopa in the treatment of parkinsonism.

MAO inhibitors: used in the treatment of depression by their action on NA metabolism in the CNS. They have widespread actions, and have hazardous interactions (see Chapter 14).

Synthesis of adrenaline

Tyrosine (which is hydroxyphenylalanine, an amino acid) is further hydroxylated by tyrosine hydroxylase to dihydroxyphenylalanine (*DOPA*). The carboxylic acid group of the alanine is removed by dopadecarboxylase, leaving the NH_2 group: *dopamine*. The beta-carbon is hydroxylated by dopamine beta-hydrolyase to form *noradrenaline*, and this further methylated to form *adrenaline* (see Fig. 10.2).

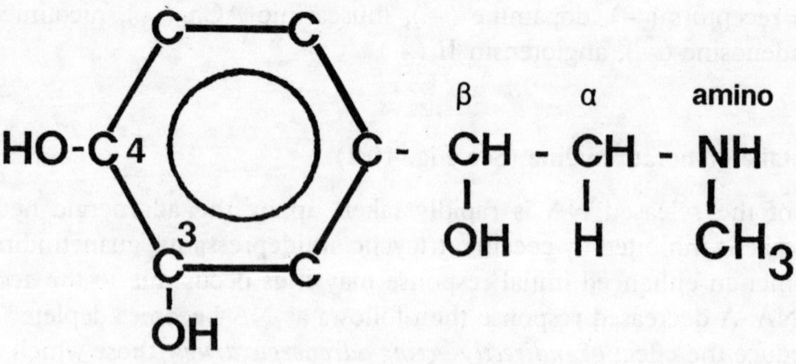

Fig. 10.2 Adrenaline.

STRUCTURE–ACTION RELATIONSHIPS

The catecholamines provide a useful example of the relationship between chemical modifications of the molecule and varying effects.

Directly-acting drugs have two OH groups on C3 and C4, as in adrenaline, NA, dopamine.

Indirectly-acting drugs have either no OH or one OH on C3 or C4: ephedrine, methamphetamine, tyramine, metaraminol.

Note:

1. An OH on the beta-carbon is necessary for a direct action.
2. A CH_3 on the alpha-carbon prevents metabolism by MAO: ephedrine, metaraminol, phenylpropylamine.
3. Substitution with larger groups on the amino position enhances beta activity: salbutamol, terbutaline, isoprenaline.

TREATMENT OF HYPERTENSION

Drugs used to control hypertension are very commonly encountered by anaesthetists: a summary of their main actions should be remembered. The following summary starts at the CNS and moves to the periphery.

1. *Centrally-acting:*
   Clonidine, an alpha$_2$ agonist, reduces sympathetic outflow.
   Methyldopa depletes noradrenaline.
   Sedatives and tranquillizers have also been used non-specifically. Reserpine was also used, depleting noradrenaline and serotonin.

2. *Ganglion blocking:*
   Hexamethonium, mecamylamine and pempidine: abandoned as they blocked both sympathetic and parasympathetic outflows.

3. *Adrenergic neurone blockers:*
Guanethidine: depletes noradrenaline.

4. *Alpha-adrenoreceptor blockers:*
Phentolamine (Rogitine), a shorter-acting drug used as a diagnostic test in, and preoperatively for, phaeochromocytoma.
Phenoxybenzamine (Dibenyline), longer-acting and used to control episodic hypertension in phaeochromocytoma. It also blocks receptors for serotonin, histamine and ACh. It blocks both neural and extraneural uptake of NA, and a beta-receptor blocker is necessary to reduce the enhanced beta-effects which result. See note at end of section.

5. *Beta-adrenoreceptor blockers:*
Propranolol (Table 10.1).

6. *Alpha and beta-adrenoreceptor blocker:*
Labetalol (Trandate).

7. *Vasodilators:*
Hydralazine (Apresoline). Bioavailability is 55%, and its direct action on vascular smooth muscle (especially coronary, cerebral, renal and splanchnic) avoids postural hypotension. Chronic dosage carries a risk of a lupus-like syndrome developing.
Prazosin (Minipress), an alpha$_1$ blocker acting mainly on arteriolar smooth muscle. Reflex tachycardia is uncommon, but postural hypotension occurs.
Debrisoquine (Declinax) interferes with NA release. It acts for 12–24 h, and may cause postural hypotension especially in the elderly.
Minoxidil (Loniten) relaxes arteriolar smooth muscle but there is a reflex increase in cardiac output, salt and water retention and renin activity. It is long-acting.
Diazoxide is a depressor of arteriolar smooth muscle. It is used intravenously for the urgent control of hypertension. Recovery begins in 10–20 min but the effects last from 3–12 h.
Indapamide (Natrilix) appears to reduce the vascular reactivity to pressor amines, and is natriuretic in the distal renal tubule.
Angiotensin-converting enzyme (ACE) inhibitors, captopril (Capoten), *enalapril* (Renitec). (See also p 121.) By suppressing angiotensin II formation they reduce blood pressure. Renin output is increased and aldosterone production falls with sodium and water loss: **hypotension during anaesthesia** can be profound and should be treated with i.v. saline.

Although not used to treat hypertension, the organic nitrates are also vasodilators: *glyceryl trinitrate* (Trinitrin, short-acting), and *isosorbide dinitrate* (Isordil, longer-acting). Used in angina pectoris, they dilate the coronary arteries, but by venodilation also reduce the preload on the heart.
Note: Vasodilators are also used to induce hypotension during anaesthesia (see below).

8. *Calcium-channel blockers* (Table 10.3)
   Verapamil (Isoptin, Cordilox, Verpamil).
   Nifedipine (Adalat).
   Diltiazem (Cardiazem).
   Felodipine (Agon).

   Note: Ca^{2+} **release in various types of muscle.** Calcium controls muscle contraction, but the three types of muscle vary in the source of Ca^{2+}.
   Skeletal muscle derives its Ca^{2+} from intracellular stores in the sarcoplasmic reticulum, release from these being triggered by Ca^{2+} entering through the transverse tubules. Hence Ca^{2+} channel blockers do not affect contraction.
   Cardiac muscle derives its Ca^{2+} both from intracellular stores (triggered by Ca^{2+} entry) and entry through Ca^{2+} channels: hence channel blockers affect contraction.
   Smooth muscle derives its Ca^{2+} from intracellular stores (triggered both by Ca^{2+} entry and cell receptors) and Ca^{2+} entering through channels. Hence channel blockers affect its contraction, but there are differences between it and cardiac muscle.

9. *Diuretic agents*
   The *thiazide* group are very commonly used, with loss of both Na^+ and K^+ following inhibition of chloride reabsorption in the ascending loop. Potassium levels may fall, with the risk of digoxin toxicity. *Frusemide* (Lasix) and *ethacrynic acid* (Edecrin) are loop diuretics of greater potency, causing potassium loss also. *Spironolactone* (Aldactone) is an aldosterone antagonist, leading to less K^+ loss.

   Note: the risk of **rebound hypertension** with possible cardiac failure or even cerebral haemorrhage can follow sudden cessation of antihypertensive drugs, especially clonidine; and *dosage should be maintained when anaesthesia is to be given.*

   It is also important to be aware that most antihypertensive agents pose a hazard during anaesthesia as they *depress the reflex responses to hypotension* which may be caused by blood loss or depression of the heart or vascular tone by anaesthetic drugs. Particular care must be taken to *restore and maintain fluid balance*. Vasodepressant drugs should be used with caution, and

Table 10.3 Calcium channel blockers

	Verapamil	Nifedipine	Diltiazem	Felodipine
Peripheral vascular resistance	- -	- - -	-	- -
Coronary vessel resistance	- -	- - -	- -	
Heart rate	+ / -	+ +	-	+
Cardiac output	+ / -	+ +	-	+
Inotropic action	- -	0	-	0
Cardiac conduction	- -	0	-	0
Contractility	-	0	-	0
t½β	8 h	4 h	6 h	25 h

sympathetic nerve block by local anaesthetic techniques used judiciously in patients who are taking antihypertensive drugs.

INDUCED HYPOTENSION

Ganglion block was originally used to achieve this. The lack of control and unpredictable offset of action subsequently led to the use of short-acting vasodilators, usually combined with the circulatory depressant effect of halothane or enflurane. More recently isoflurane has become favoured because it lowers the systemic vascular resistance without decreasing the cardiac output, unlike the other volatile agents.

Sodium nitroprusside (SNP, Nipride)

SNP directly depresses vascular tone, lowering arterial and venous pressures. Its action is extremely brief. Exact control of dose-rate is essential (see below). It is, therefore, given only by infusion: the rate is from $1-12 \ \mu gkg^{-1}min^{-1}$.

Metabolism and hazards

1. It is rapidly converted to cyanide by haemoglobin and free sulphydryl groups. The cyanide is converted by the hepatic enzyme rhodanase to cyanate which is excreted by the kidney. *If dosage is exceeded, cyanide can accumulate,* forming cyanmethaemoglobin and combining with cytochrome oxidase with consequent signs of toxicity: metabolic acidosis, increased venous PO_2. Recommended treatment: slow i.v. injection of sodium nitrite 3% up to 10 ml, followed by sodium thiosulphate, 12.5 g in 50 ml 5% dextrose over 10 min. The nitrite forms methaemoglobin which removes the cyanide from the cytochrome oxidase, and thiosulphate converts cyanide to cyanate.

2. Hydroxocobalamin (Vitamin B12) has been used prophylactically to avoid toxicity by combining with cyanide to form cyanocobalamin.

3. *If a patient is resistant to the hypotensive action, it is important not to exceed the limited dose-rate, but to use other methods to reduce the blood pressure.*

4. SNP is rapidly *decomposed by light:* containers should be masked.

Glyceryl trinitrate

Decreases venous and arteriolar tone resulting in increased pooling and decreased preload. Its $t\frac{1}{2}\beta$ is 1–4 min. It is given as 100 $\mu g/ml$ in 5% glucose or 0.9% saline. Initial dose rate is 5 $\mu gkg^{-1}min^{-1}$. Resistant patients may need a stronger solution and dose increments of 10 $\mu gkg^{-1}min^{-1}$. The drug is strongly adsorbed to PVC tubing: special i.v. sets are available to avoid this. The drug is stable in dilute solution and not affected by light. A precise means of regulating the dose-rate is necessary. The metabolites appear to be inactive.

Trimetaphan

Blocks sympathetic and parasympathetic ganglia, releases histamine and directly reduces peripheral vascular tone: a compensatory tachycardia may limit the fall in blood pressure. The response is unpredictable: acute tolerance may occur. Conversely, prolonged hypotension (possibly related to histamine release) may follow its use.

It is metabolized by plasma cholinesterase although it is not an ester.

NOTES

1. The desensitization of adrenoreceptors

Small amounts of NA are continually released at sympathetic junctional tissue, similar to the release of quanta of ACh at the neuromuscular junction (with miniature end-plate potentials). This NA appears to maintain a state of desensitization. When NA is depleted (by guanethidine) or is suppressed (by sympathectomy), the response to circulating NA or directly-acting sympathomimetics is greatly enhanced.

2. The stability of adrenaline in solution

Dilute solutions of adrenaline rapidly oxidize in light and air unless stabilized by a reducing agent (bisulphite) or by acidification.

3. Phaeochromocytoma

This chromaffin tumour releases NA predominantly, with episodic hypertension and reduced circulating volume. An alpha-blocker (phenoxybenzamine: 1–3 mg/kg) controls the alpha effects, but blocks the feedback suppression of NA release, with enhanced beta-effects. A beta-adrenoreceptor blocker must also be given, and the reduced circulating blood volume restored. At operation NA may be released when the tumour is handled, and nitroprusside can be used to control the blood pressure without the risk of postoperative hypotension.

Metyrosine (alpha-methyltyrosine), an inhibitor of tyrosine hydroxylase, has been used to depress catechol synthesis before operation.

11. Antiarrhythmic drugs and digoxin

NORMAL RHYTHM

The membrane potential in heart muscle and Purkinje fibres alters in five phases: *phase 0* is the period of rapid Na^+ entry; *phases 1* and *2* are the plateau of the action potential associated with electromechanical coupling and Ca^{2+} entry; *phase 3* is repolarization and K^+ exit, and *phase 4* is the spontaneous depolarization related to pacemaker activity. The sinoatrial (SA) and atrioventricular (AV) nodes do not have a phase 2 plateau, and depolarization during phase 4 is faster (see Fig. 11.1).

Arrhythmias are due to abnormal impulse formation and/or abnormal propagation.

THE ANTIARRHYTHMIC DRUGS

The Vaughan-Williams and Singh classification:

Class I
Act by blocking fast Na^+ current (slowing phase 0 depolarization).
   a. Slow rate of depolarization and prolong action potential: *quinidine, procainamide, disopyramide.*

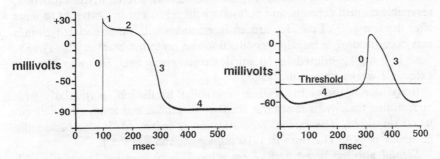

Fig 11.1 Cardiac action potentials. Left Cardiac muscle: phase 0 is the fast inward current of Na^+, phase 2 the slow inward current of Ca^{2+}, and phase 3 the slow outward current of K^+. Right SA and AV nodes: phase 4 is an outward current of K^+ and slow inward current of Na^+ and Ca^{2+}, phase 0 is the fast inward current of Na^+, and phase 3 the slow outward current of K^+.

   b. Slow rate of depolarization in ischaemic cells, shorten action potential: *lignocaine, mexilitine, tocainamide.*
   c. Depolarization rate markedly slowed with QRS prolongation: *flecainide.*

Class II

Block the effect of catecholamines. Beta-adrenoreceptor blockers: *propranolol, atenolol, metoprolol.*

Class III

Lengthen the action potential, prolonging phase 3 repolarization. *Amiodarone, bretylium, sotalol.*

Class IV

Calcium channel blockers. *Verapamil, diltiazem.* (Nifedipine acts only on non-cardiac smooth muscle and is not an antiarrhythmic.)

Notes on antiarrhythmic drugs

Quinidine is well absorbed orally, PPB 55%, t½β 8 h. A test dose of 200 mg monitored with ECG should be given to detect idiosyncrasy, with depressed conduction leading to asystole. Quinidine reduces the excitability, automaticity and conduction velocity in the atrium, AV node and ventricle, increasing the duration of the action potential and effective refractory period. The slope of phase 0 of the node is decreased, as is the phase 4 of Purkinje fibres.

Disopyramide (Norpace, Rythmodan), t½β 4–10 h. Has local anaesthetic properties and marked anticholinergic effects. Its actions are similar to quinidine.

Beta-adrenoreceptor blockers (See Table 10.1).

Amiodarone is an extremely effective drug both for acute or chronic control of arrhythmias. It is also a peripheral vasodilator. Chronic usage is associated with serious toxicity: hepatic dysfunction, altered thyroid function, reversible corneal deposits, and pulmonary fibrosis occur in 5–10% of patients after the first year of use. Hazardous interactions with other antiarrhythmics may occur leading to impaired conduction and profound bradycardia. The i.v. dose is 5 mg/kg diluted in 50 ml dextrose, given over 60 min. The t½β exceeds 2 weeks after oral dosage.

Bretylium is useful in treating ventricular fibrillation, particularly with bupivacaine toxicity. It raises the fibrillary threshold and lowers the defibrillation threshold. The rate of repolarization is increased. It also blocks the re-uptake of NA. The dose is 5–10 mg/kg i.v. and t½β 7.5 h.

Sotalol also has beta-adrenoreceptor blocking properties. The t½β is 13 h and the loading dose is 1 mg/kg.

Verapamil and related drugs: see Chapter 10.

DIGOXIN

Not included in the Vaughan-Williams classification. Widely used in atrial fibrillation and cardiac failure.

Pharmacokinetics

70% absorbed orally; PPB 23%. Plasma $t\frac{1}{2}\beta$ is proportional to glomerular filtration rate: normally 36 h, 37% being excreted each day. In old age, $t\frac{1}{2}\beta$ increases to 50 h due to glomerular loss; and in anuria to > 100 h. Tissue binding is extensive: myocardial/plasma ratio is 30:1 and increases with hypokalaemia or hyponatraemia.

Pharmacodynamics

Increases availability of Ca^{2+} in sarcoplasmic reticulum, promoting excitation/contraction coupling. Increases vagal tone by sensitizing carotid baroreceptors. Decreases conduction velocity. In *toxic doses* it may lead to *heart block or ventricular fibrillation* (by shortening the ventricular refractory period and enhancing subsidiary pacemakers).

Factors enhancing toxicity

1. *Hypokalaemia,* mainly related to K^+-losing diuretics. *Note:* phenytoin is effective in treating digoxin-induced arrhythmias when there is hypokalemia.
2. *Overdosage or renal failure:* dose should be related to creatinine clearance.
3. *Drugs which alter kinetics:* quinidine, verapamil reduce renal clearance, quinidine reduces the volume of distribution, amiodarone enhances the plasma level.
4. *Low Mg^{2+}, high Ca^{2+}, hypoxia, myocardial ischaemia, acidosis, hypothyroidism.*

Toxic signs and symptoms

1. Cardiac arrhythmias
2. CNS: blurred vision, coloured vision, headache, drowsiness
3. Gut: nausea, vomiting, pain
4. Gynaecomastia
5. Thrombocytopenia.

Digitalizing dose

- Orally: 0.5 mg then 0.25 mg 6-hourly up to 1.5 mg.

- Maintenance: 0.125–0.5 mg daily: it takes 7 days (5 half-lives) to reach a steady state.
- Intravenously: 0.25 mg by slow injection, repeated 4–6 hourly up to 1.0 mg.
- Therapeutic plasma level: 1.3–2.6 nanomole/litre.

12. Diuretics

Under normal physiological conditions, the reabsorption of various ions and water is effected by certain specific parts of the nephron (see below). Diuretics act by targeting these specific areas.

Functions of the nephron

    a. Proximal convoluted tubule: active reabsorption of Na^+, phosphate, bicarbonate, glucose, amino acids. Passive reabsorption of Cl^-, water.

    b. Descending limb: passive reabsorption of water.

    c. Ascending limb: active reabsorption of Cl^-, passive reabsorption of Na^+.

    d. Distal convoluted tubule: active reabsorption of Na^+ (and some K^+ in states of severe depletion), passive reabsorption of Cl^-, excretion of K^+, active and passive H^+ transfer.

    e. Collecting duct: passive water reabsorption (via antidiuretic hormone), active Na^+ reabsorption (via aldosterone), active and passive excretion of K^+ and H^+.

Urea can passively diffuse from the papillary part to the medullary interstitium.

Osmotic diuretics

Mannitol (Osmitrol): dilates the afferent arteriole, raising glomerular pressure and renal plasma flow. It reduces water reabsorption in the proximal tubule. Dose: 0.5 g/kg.

Loop diuretics

Frusemide (Lasix) inhibits active Na^+ and Cl^- reabsorption in the medullary and cortical segments of the ascending limb. K^+ loss increases due to increased flow of water and Na^+ though the distal tubule. **Ethacrynic acid** (Edecril) inhibits salt and water reabsorption mainly in the ascending limb, producing an iso-osmotic urine. **Bumetanide** (Burinex) also inhibits Na^+

reabsorption in the ascending limb, an action similar to the now obsolescent organomercurials.

Sulphonamide derivatives: the thiazides

Chlorothiazide (Chlotride), hydrochlorothiazide (Dichlotride), bendrofluazide (Aprinox), cyclopenthiazide (Navidrex), methychlothiazide (Enduron), chlorthalidone (Hygroton), indapamide (Natrilix). Inhibit tubular electrolyte reabsorption and cause a *passive K^+ loss* in the distal nephron. Mg^{2+} and $HCO3^-$ are also lost. Some inhibit carbonic anhydrase, with loss of bicarbonate and phosphate: acetazolamide (Diamox) is a powerful inhibitor and is used to lower the intraocular pressure.

Aldosterone antagonists

Na^+ reabsorption in the distal tubule is controlled by aldosterone. Spironolactone (Aldactone) is a competitive antagonist: Na^+ is lost and K^+ conserved. K^+ retention makes this drug useful in hepatic cirrhosis and in those receiving digoxin where low K^+ levels may enhance toxicity.

Non-competitive inhibitors of Na^+ reabsorption in the distal tubule

Triamterene (Dytac), amiloride (Midamor, Moduretic). These are K^+ conserving diuretics as K^+ is not lost in exchange for Na^+.

13. Inorganic ions: Na^+; K^+, Ca^{2+}, Mg^{2+}, Li^+

SODIUM

The chief extracellular cation

Small changes in Na^+ produce little change in excitable tissues. A rise results in fluid retention via the antidiuretic hormone: a sharp rise (e.g. following high Na^+ in enemas in infants) may cause convulsions. Na^+ can also be given in high dosage inadvertently in hypertonic bicarbonate (treating acidosis), or in Na^+ salts of penicillin.

A fall follows excessive Na^+-free i.v. fluids, excessive sweating or inappropriate antidiuretic hormone secretion (due to prolonged raised intrathoracic pressure from IPPV, or from drugs: tricyclics, thiazides, some cytotoxics). A profound fall (to 110 mmol/l or less) may cause intracranial haemorrhage. This should be treated promptly but cautiously with 1.8% saline infusion or by increasing the renal free water excretion with Lasix. There is a risk of pontine myelinosis with too rapid correction of Na^+.

Therapeutic use is most commonly isotonic saline (150 mmol/l) or 4% glucose/0.18% saline (30 mmol/l) solution, or compound sodium lactate (130 mmol/l).

POTASSIUM

The chief intracellular cation

Only 2% of K^+ is extracellular: a normal plasma level (3.5–5 mmol/l) may be found despite severe depletion of intracellular K^+. K^+ readily enters cells, especially under the influence of insulin and glucose, so that an intracellular depletion can rapidly lead to plasma hypokalaemia.

Heart

Raised K^+ depresses conductivity and arrests the heart in diastole. Low concentration leads to asystolic arrest or ventricular failure (VF), especially with digoxin or raised Ca^{2+}.

ECG: <3.0 mmol/l depresses S-T segment, flattens T wave, large U waves. Q-T prolonged, arrhythmias. >5.0 mmol/l leads to augmented T waves (which can be confused with posterior myocardial infarct or pericarditis), atrial arrest, widening of QRS (see Fig. 13.1).

Neuromuscular junction

Raised K⁺ moves resting potential towards threshold: depolarization occurs more readily, ***antagonising non-depolarization block.***

Lowered K⁺ hyperpolarizes the postjunctional membrane, ***increasing non-depolarizing block.*** The ED_{50} for dTC has been reported to fall from 0.5 µmol/l at 5.0 mmol/l K⁺ to 0.2 µmol/l at 2.0 mmol/l, experimentally.

In *familial periodic paralysis* K⁺ falls with marked muscle weakness.

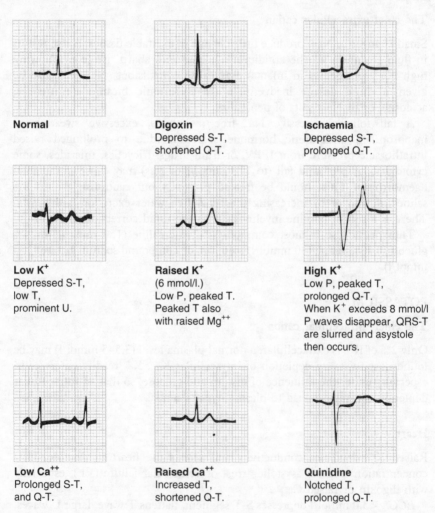

Normal

Digoxin
Depressed S-T,
shortened Q-T.

Ischaemia
Depressed S-T,
prolonged Q-T.

Low K⁺
Depressed S-T,
low T,
prominent U.

Raised K⁺
(6 mmol/l.)
Low P, peaked T.
Peaked T also
with raised Mg⁺⁺

High K⁺
Low P, peaked T,
prolonged Q-T.
When K⁺ exceeds 8 mmol/l
P waves disappear, QRS-T
are slurred and asystole
then occurs.

Low Ca⁺⁺
Prolonged S-T,
and Q-T.

Raised Ca⁺⁺
Increased T,
shortened Q-T.

Quinidine
Notched T,
prolonged Q-T.

Fig. 13.1 ECG changes.

Gut

Hypokalaemia leads to atony.

K^+ kinetics

Body content is 3700 mmol/70 kg. Daily requirement for i.v. therapy is 1 mmol/kg (3 g/70 kg).

Maximum infusion rate is 0.5 mmol kg^{-1} h^{-1}. Hypertonic K^+ solutions are very irritant to veins.

Causes of depletion: K^+-deficient i.v. fluids, diarrhoea, small bowel fistulae, diabetic ketoacidosis, aldosteronism, thiazide and loop diuretics. Care must be taken to avoid hypokalaemia during resuscitation of diabetic acidosis and pyloric stenosis.

Hyperkalaemia is treated by inducing alkalaemia i.e. bicarbonate infusion and hyperventilation. Glucose and insulin also lower the serum potassium although not as quickly. Calcium may reverse acute arrhythmias. It is a hazard if suxamethonium is given to patients with burns or denervation injuries.

CALCIUM

Plasma level 2.1–2.8 mmol/l, 55% being ionized. Intracellular level 0.001 mmol/l. Ca^{2+} entry through calcium channels is involved in most cellular activity: it becomes attached to calmodulin in the release of hormones and transmitters, to troponin in the contraction of myofibrils. It is part of the blood coagulation cascade. Its role in cardiac automaticity is given in Chapter 11, in muscle contraction in Chapter 8.

Hypercalcaemia is seen in hyperparathyroidism and Vitamin D intoxications. It results in skeletal muscle weakness, and ECG changes (increased T wave, shortened Q-T interval, see Fig. 13.1).

Hypocalcaemia is seen in hypoparathyroidism and renal insufficiency. Skeletal muscle cramps and tetany occur, and cardiac output falls. ECG has prolongation of both S-T and Q-T intervals (see also Fig. 13.1). Treatment of hypocalcaemia is 10 ml 10% calcium chloride (27 mg Ca^{2+}/ml) given slowly or diluted as it is injurious to veins. Calcium gluconate is also used but is less bioavailable: the 10% solution contains 9 mg Ca^{2+}/ml.

MAGNESIUM

Plasma level 0.7–1.05 mmol/l, 66% as Mg^{2+}; 60% is in bone, 30% in muscle, 9% in other soft tissues, 1% in blood. It forms Mg-ATP and Mg-NAD complex in mitochondria, activating ATPase which is essential for the Na^+/K^+ pump. It is essential for enzymes which use ATP and those which transfer phosphate groups (formation of cyclic AMP from ATP). It has an important role via magnesium-dependent ATPase which effects calcium re-uptake into sarcoplasmic reticulum during muscle activity. Mg^{2+} is essential for the release of parathyroid hormone and is a cofactor for its effect on bone, kidney and gut.

Raised Mg^{2+}. In renal failure, adrenocortical insufficiency, excessive intake, lithium therapy and iatrogenically in the treatment of pre-eclampsia. *CNS:* drowsiness, hyporeflexia. Above 5 mmol/l respiratory depression occurs, above 10 mmol/l, coma. *NMJ:* antagonizes Ca^{2+}, reducing ACh release and excitability. Enhances non-depolarizing neuromuscular blockade. *CVS:* vasodilation and hypotension. *ECG:* prolonged P-R and Q-T intervals, slows SA node impulse rate. Heart arrests in diastole.

Low Mg^{2+}: Always accompanied by low Ca^{2+}, and often hypokalemia if associated with diuretic treatment. It is due to deficient intake (especially in alcoholics), decreased intestinal absorption or increased loss (prolonged diarrhoea, renal tubular dysfunction, diuresis, hyperaldosteronism and ethanol toxicity). *CNS:* apathy, depression, anxiety, hallucinations, convulsions. *NMJ:* tetany. *CVS:* hypertension, vasoconstriction, increased myocardial excitability. Enhances digoxin toxicity. Treatment: 0.5 mmol/kg of magnesium sulphate over 3 h then 0.75 mmol/kg over 21 h.

LITHIUM

Exchanges with Na^+ at a cellular level. Used in manic-depressive psychosis, with careful plasma monitoring as it can damage the kidney resulting in reduced glomerular filtration and nephrotic syndrome.

It is filtered completely by the glomeruli but 80% reabsorbed. Reabsorption occurs in the proximal tubule, although it is linked to that of Na^+, it is reabsorbed preferentially.

14. Psychoactive drugs and anticonvulsants

ANTIPSYCHOTIC DRUGS

Phenothiazines

These are used extensively in psychiatry, pain control, anaesthetic premedication and also prescribed as antiemetics. There are three groups, based on the substitution on the nitrogen atom:

a. aliphatic: chlorpromazine (Largactil), promethazine (Phenergan), trimeprazine (Vallergan)
b. piperidine: thioridazine (Melleril)
c. piperazine: prochlorperazine (Stemetil), trifluoperazine (Stelazine).

They are associated with a wide range of *side-effects,* especially with prolonged dosage. Of particular importance is *cholestatic jaundice* with chlorpromazine, and *extrapyramidal side-effects* with the piperazine derivatives. The latter may be seen early in their use, and limits the use of prochlorperazine as an antiemetic.

Pharmacokinetics

Distributed widely and are metabolized. Some metabolites are removed slowly.

Pharmacodynamics

CNS

Depression. The antipsychotic action is due to blocking of dopamine receptors. D_1 receptors are related to adenyl cyclase stimulation, and may modulate the behavioural and biochemical effects of D_2 receptors (which inhibit adenyl cyclase).

Some dopamine pathways and the effects of block are:

1. nigrostriatal – extrapyramidal effects
2. tuberoinfundibular – antiemetic
3. mesolimbic – ?antipsychotic.

139

Promethazine is a hypnotic. All the common members are antiemetics, prochlorperazine being the most potent. Temperature regulation is depressed, aiding the induction of hypothermia.

Extrapyramidal side-effects

Parkinsonism is the commonest one reported. There are decreased body movements, mask-like face, increased muscle tone and tremor. *Benztropine* (Cogentin) or *benzhexol* (Artane) are antidotes. *Acute dystonia:* muscle spasms; akathesia (restlessness) and tardive dyskinesia (abnormal involuntary movements) are also described.

Autonomic nervous system

Promethazine is an anticholinergic and dries salivary secretions. It is also a potent antihistamine and local anaesthetic.
Chlorpromazine has mild antiadrenergic and anticholinergic actions.
  CVS: reduces blood pressure mainly by central effects on CNS.
  Skeletal muscle: Non-depolarizing neuromuscular block is slightly enhanced, probably by the anticholinergic action.
  Endocrine: ACTH release is decreased and the response to stress lessened by chlorpromazine. This is part of the basis of 'neuroleptic' techniques.
  Liver: cholestatic jaundice may follow prolonged treatment with chlorpromazine.
  Other complications: skin rashes, bone marrow depression, gynaecomastia, galactorrhoea, amenorrhoea, photosensitivity.

Butyrophenones

Droperidol (Droleptan) is the most commonly used member.
  Pharmacokinetics: t½β 127 min; Vd 103 l; clearance 732 ml/min.
  Pharmacodynamics: It is a potent sedative, antiemetic and antiadrenergic.
  Side-effects: Patients may appear tranquil but later complain of dysphoria with feelings of anxiety and terror which they have been unable to express. It should be avoided in patients with a history of depression. A very small dose (1 mg) reduces the incidence of dysphoria but remains effective as an antiemetic.

ANTIDEPRESSANTS

Tricyclics

Doxepin (Sinequan) and dothiepin (Prothiaden) are the safest members. Others include amitriptyline (Tryptanol, Laroxyl, Mutabon), trimipramine (Surmontil), imipramine (Tofranil) and nortriptyline (Allegron, Aventyl).

Mianserin, a *tetracyclic*, is also used. It is less toxic to the heart in overdose, and has very little anticholinergic action (Elliot-Baker et al 1990, Tiller 1990).

Pharmacodynamics

Tricyclic antidepressants interfere with noradrenaline re-uptake, enhancing NA's actions. Anticholinergic actions result in a dry mouth, blurred vision and urinary retention. Antidepressant effect is delayed: single doses may produce sedation.

Toxic effects

In overdose severe cardiac arrhythmias occur. These are difficult to treat and may lead to ventricular fibrillation.

Special note: hazard with MAO inhibitors

The accumulated noradrenaline occurring with MAO inhibitors and the reduced re-uptake of noradrenaline with tricyclics can combine to give convulsions, hyperpyrexia and hypertension.

Monoamine oxidase inhibitors (MAOIs)

Pharmacodynamics

Type A MAO occurs in cells which release NA as transmitter (parts of the brain and sympathetic synapses). It acts on polar aromatic amines (serotonin, NA). Type B is seen in the gut (where it metabolizes non-polar aromatic monoamines in foodstuffs) and the liver.

MAOIs include tranylcypromine (Parnate, Parstelin), isocarboxazid (Marplan), phenelzine (Nardil). MAOIs also inhibit other liver microsomal enzymes (diamine oxidase, choline oxidase and amphetamine oxidase).

Their use results in:

1. **Rise of concentration of amines** in brain, heart and gut, due to decreased breakdown and increased storage. The therapeutic effects in the CNS appear to be related to the increased NA and serotonin (5-HT). They are profound suppressors of REM sleep.

2. **Increased nervous activity.** Chlorpromazine has been used to control this by antagonizing the effects of the serotonin, NA and dopamine which accumulate.

3. Inhibition of MAO in the gut. Tyramine (in cheese, meat extracts, beer and many foods) is no longer metabolized, and its absorption results in the release of NA (it is an indirect adrenergic agonist) and the risk of a hypertensive crisis. Fruits and caffeine-containing drinks may produce bizarre

effects due to the absorption of unchanged dopamine, tyramine and serotonin. (See also *Interactions* below.)

4. *Possible side-effects and toxic effects:*
   i.   acute hepatic necrosis
   ii. red-green colour blindness
   iii. anaemia, thrombocytopaenia
   iv. orthostatic hypotension
   v.   hypoglycaemia
   vi. tremor, insomnia.

Interactions

These may be classed as:

1. Major importance:

   - Pethidine: agitation, headache, blood pressure rises or falls, rigidity, convulsions, coma, hyperpyrexia
   - Tricyclic antidepressants: delirium, seizures, tremors, hypertonia, hyperpyrexia
   - Levodopa: hypertension (carbidopa inhibits this response)
   - Indirectly-acting sympathomimetic drugs (ephedrine, amphetamine, phenylpropanolamine, methylphenidate): hypertension with headache, chest pain, tachycardia, stroke, heart failure or convulsions, hyperpyrexia, vomiting. *Note:* phenylpropanolamine in proprietary nasal decongestants can release NA. Hence this non-prescription drug can be hazardous with MAOIs.
   - Mixed (directly- and indirectly-acting) sympathomimetic drugs (metaraminol, dopamine, phenylephrine): as for indirect group above
   - Dietary group.

2. Minor importance:

   - Morphine: enhanced depression
   - Inhalation anaesthetics: may be enhanced
   - Phenothiazines: enhanced.

3. No interaction:

   - Local anaesthetics, antihistamines, beta-adrenoreceptor blockers, benzodiazepines, directly-acting sympathomimetics (adrenaline particularly).

Note

1. *The prolonged duration of effect means that drugs must be withdrawn 10–14 days before elective surgery if risks are anticipated.*
2. *Directly-acting sympathomimetic drugs are not enhanced by MAOIs: adrenaline, NA, dopamine, methoxamine.*

Other antidepressants

1. Serotonin-uptake inhibitors may give a more specific means of treatment: fluoxetine, fluvoxamine and sertraline have been developed.
2. Lithium carbonate is also used. It is toxic in overdose, making blood assays mandatory.
3. Amphetamine and its derivatives have been withdrawn because of dependence and abuse. Illegal manufacture is frequently reported in the media.

ANTICONVULSANTS (See Table 14.1)

All the drugs mentioned in Table 14.1 are used for convulsive seizures except: *Clonazepam* (myoclonic seizures) and *ethosuximide* (absence seizures).

Note: For immediate control of convulsions, especially those due to toxic effects of local anaesthetics, thiopentone (1–2 mg/kg), diazepam (0.1–0.2 mg/kg) or midazolam (0.25–0.05 mg/kg) are very effective.

Table 14.1 Anticonvulsants

Drug	$mgkg^{-1}day^{-1}$	$t_{1/2}$	Concentration	Side-effects
Phenytoin (Dilantin)	4–8	24 h	40–80 µmol/l	Gingival hyperplasia, hirsutism
Phenobarbitone	2–5	3–4 days	45–110 µmol/l	Mental slowing
Primidone (Mysoline)	5–20	3–12 h	25–70 µmol/l	Acts as phenobarbitone
Carbamazepine (Tegretol)	5–20	36 h	25–70 µmol/l	Rash, drowsiness
Clonazepam (Rivotril)	0.05–0.20	24 h	0.02–2.20 nm/l	Drowsiness, fatigue, ataxia, irritability
Ethosuximide (Zarontin)	15–60	2–3 days	300–700 µmol/l	Anorexia, nausea, vomiting, rash
Sodium valproate (Epilim)	10–40	8–10 h	350–700 µmol/l	Vomiting, tremor, rarely liver toxicity

FURTHER READING

Elliot-Baker S J, Singh B S 1990 What has happened to the new antidepressant drugs? Medical Journal of Australia 152: 150–152
Tiller J W G 1990 A review of anti-anxiety agents. Medical Journal of Australia 151: 697–701

15. Adrenocortical drugs

MAJOR HORMONES

1. Glucocorticoids: predominantly cortisol (20 mg/day)
2. Mineralocorticoids: predominantly aldosterone (125 µg/day)
3. Androgens (20 mg/day), oestrogens a trace.

Cortisol

Cortisol production is controlled by *corticotrophin*. Corticotrophin is produced by the anterior pituitary in response to:

1. *Stress:* stimuli from the cortex pass to the hypothalamus where corticotrophin-releasing factor (CRF), a polypeptide, is released. Morphine blocks this release. CRF is carried by the hypophyseal portal system to the pituitary gland.
2. *Feedback:* cortisol reduces the response of the hypothalamus, anterior pituitary and the adrenal cortex.

In *acute stress* up to 300 mg/day may be released. Diurnal variation: the highest level occurs in the early morning, and there is a slow decrease during the evening. There is no storage of cortisol.

Actions of cortisol

1. *Gluconeogenesis:* excess produces hyperglycaemia, impaired glucose tolerance with glycosuria, insulin resistance and increased liver glycogen.
2. *Protein metabolism:* excess induces a negative nitrogen balance with muscle wasting, increased urinary creatinine and uric acid, retarded growth, osteoporosis.
3. *Lipid metabolism:* increased deposition of fat in the trunk and face (moon-face), increased serum triglycerides.
4. *Diuresis:* by impairing the shift of water into cells.
5. *Blood cells:* anti-inflammatory and immunosuppressive; decrease in eosinophils and lymphocytes, increase in neutrophils and erythrocytes. Response of B and T cells to antigens is suppressed.

6. *Gastric acidity and pepsin production:* increase.

7. *Bone:* cartilage development is impaired, calcium absorption from the gut and deposition in bone are reduced and increased urinary loss of calcium and phosphate occurs.

8. *Mood:* excess may lead to the development of psychosis.

9. *Resistance to infection:* cortisol may reduce the tissue response to injury.

10. *Excretion:* sodium and chloride excretion decreased, potassium excretion increased.

Aldosterone

Aldosterone production is under the influence of:

1. *Angiotensin II:* derived from angiotensin I by renin, it enhances aldosterone production.
2. *Vascular volume:* a decrease due to haemorrhage, sodium restriction or dehydration increases aldosterone production.
3. *Potassium* level in the blood.

Actions of aldosterone

Sodium is conserved in exchange for potassium amd hydrogen ions, leading to hypertension, hypokalaemia and muscle weakness.

Corticosteroid drugs

These drugs vary with respect to their duration of action and dynamics, potency, anti-inflammatory and salt-retaining efficacy. These properties determine the therapeutic uses of these drugs (see Table 15.1).

Note: Etomidate and the antifungal drug *ketoconazole* both interfere with cortisol production by inhibiting 11-beta-hydroxylase acting on 11-deoxycortisol, and have been associated with adrenocortical insufficiency.

Synacthen stimulates the cortex directly to produce cortisol and aldosterone.

Replacement therapy

In Addison's disease, hypopituitarism or after adrenalectomy. Basal requirement is cortisone 20–30 mg/day, orally or i.m., rising to 300 mg in stress. Hydrocortisone hemisuccinate 100 mg can be given i.v. in emergency; it must be repeated 12-hourly.

Therapeutic actions

1. to suppress inflammation in rheumatoid arthritis and lupus erythematosus

Table 15.1 Steroid drugs (Anti-inflammatory activity and salt retention are comparative potencies, where hydrocortisone = 1)

	Dose equivalent	Anti-inflammatory	Salt retention	Uses
Glucocorticoid				
Short-acting				
Cortisone	20 mg	0.8	0.8	Standard replacement
Hydrocortisone	25 mg	1.0	1.0	Emergency replacement
Prednisone	5 mg	4.0	0.3	Cytotoxic therapy
Prednisolone	5 mg	5.0	0.3	Asthma
Medium-acting				
Triamcinolone	4 mg	5.0	0	Dermatology
Long-acting				
Betamethasone	0.60 mg	30.0	0	Suppress ACTH production
Dexamethasone	0.75 mg	30.0	0	Prevents cerebral oedema after injury or surgery
Mineralocorticoid				
Fludrocortisone	200 µg	10.0	250	Used with glucocorticoid to reduce Na$^+$ loss

2. to suppress an allergic response in asthma or drug reactions
3. to reduce lymphocyte numbers in leukaemia
4. in the management of autoimmune diseases
5. to reduce cerebral oedema after injury.

Adverse effects

1. infection may be masked
2. osteoporosis
3. peptic ulceration
4. muscle weakness
5. diabetes mellitus
6. intracranial hypertension
7. psychosis
8. retarded growth in children
9. round, red face, striae, weight gain
10. oedema, potassium loss, hypertension
11. hirsutism, acne
12. raised intraocular pressure
13. adrenocortical atrophy and acute insufficiency.

If more than 2 g cortisone (or equivalent) has been given over an extended course (several weeks), adrenocortical depression may develop and last up to 3 months. A challenge with metyrapone (Metopirone), which interferes with cortisol production, will test the ability of the pituitary to produce ACTH and the adrenal cortical response to it. A normal response is measured by raised excretion of cortisol precursors. If the response indicates cortical depression, prophylactic hydrocortisone is given: 100 mg i.v. preoperatively and 50 mg i.v. 6-hourly, decreasing over 3–5 days, depending on the severity of the surgery.

Note: Acute insufficiency is indistinguishable from hypovolaemic hypotension.

16. Histamine, antihistamine and prostaglandins

HISTAMINE

An autocoid which is released from mast cells and basophil leucocytes in response to:

1. injury,
2. normal dosage of some drugs (tubocurarine, morphine), or
3. as part of anaphylactic and anaphylactoid reactions.

Histamine is very widely distributed in the body, and some tissues have a very high turnover. Following an immune reaction, the blood level of histamine is found to be greatly increased. If a second exposure to the allergen occurs circulatory depression may result from the high histamine level.

Pharmacodynamics

Histamine₁ (H₁) receptors are present on smooth muscle of bronchi and gut, mediating bronchoconstriction and contraction. They also slow AV conduction in the heart and vasoconstrict the coronary vessels.

Histamine₂ (H₂) receptors regulate gastric secretion, and increase heart rate. They also increase cardiac contractility and dilate the coronary vessels.

Both receptors are involved in vasodilation and hypotension, and capillary dilation and increased permeability: a decrease in systemic vascular resistance (by up to 80%) may occur during immune reactions. Treatment of immune reactions should include H_1 and H_2 blockers and blood volume expansion.

Histamine also releases NA from the sympathetic nervous system, and adrenaline and NA from the suprarenal glands, causing increased myocardial contractility and arrhythmias.

HISTAMINE₁ BLOCKING DRUGS: THE 'ANTIHISTAMINES'

There are many of these, with similar actions. Promethazine (Phenergan) is used in anaesthesia; pheniramine (Avil) and its derivatives, diphenhydramine (Benadryl) and trimeprazine (Vallergan) are also widely used. Later additions are astemizole (which does not enter the CNS) and terfenadine.

Pharmacodynamics

Antagonism of bronchoconstriction, bowel contraction, vasoconstriction and capillary permeability. Reversal of the effects of histamine which has already been released does not occur. They also cause sedation, and have anticholinergic and local anaesthetic actions (especially promethazine).

Side-effects include excessive drowsiness, dryness of the mouth, hypotension and histamine release.

Promethazine is long-acting, with antiemetic, anticholinergic, tranquillizing and hypnotic actions. It enhances the effects of anaesthetics, analgesics and other hypnotics. It is a phenothiazine.

Trimeprazine, another phenothiazine, has antipruritic and sedative effects and has been used as a sedative in children.

HISTAMINE$_2$ BLOCKING DRUGS

Used very widely in the treatment of peptic ulceration and to reduce gastric acidity in anaesthesia.

Cimetidine (Tagamet) was the first drug reported. In a 300 mg dose it will raise the gastric pH to >2.5 in 85% of patients, and reduce gastric content.

Pharmacokinetics: well absorbed orally, 22% plasma protein-bound. Rapidly excreted by the kidney (60% in 2.5 h): dosage is reduced if creatinine clearance is impaired.

Pharmacodynamics: specific competitive histamine antagonism.

Side-effects: hypotension, arrhythmias and cardiac arrest have occurred after i.v. use. Confusion, particularly in the elderly. Gynaecomastia may occur.

Interactions arise from its *inhibition of cytochrome P450* in the liver, enhancing the effects of many drugs which are metabolized by this: warfarin, propranolol, lignocaine, phenytoin.

Ranitidine (Zantac) is also a selective competitive antagonist at the H$_2$ receptor. Bioavailability is 50% with about 15% PPB; 40% is excreted in the urine in 24 h, and dosage is reduced with impaired creatinine clearance. It does not inhibit cytochrome P450. Central nervous and cardiovascular system side-effects are less likely to occur than with cimetidine.

Famotidine (Pepcidine) is similar. Bioavailability is 45%. The kidney excretes 65% and the remainder is metabolized: dosage is reduced in renal impairment. It is claimed that side-effects are even less common than with ranitidine.

PROSTAGLANDINS

These are derived from membrane phospholipids which produce arachidonic acid by phospholipase A$_2$. The next step may be catalysis by lipoxygenase to produce leukotrienes and SRS-A (slow-reacting substance), two inflammatory autacoids; or by prostaglandin synthetase (cyclo-oxygenase) to form cyclic peroxides (prostaglandin G_2 and H_2).

In platelets, thromboxane synthetase next produces thromboxanes (TXA_2 and TXB_2). Other cells convert the cyclic peroxides to prostaglandin PGD_2, PGE_2 and $PGF_{2\alpha}$. In vascular endothelium, prostacylin synthetase produces prostacyclin (PGI_2).

The prostaglandins have a wide range of activity in tissues. They have very short half-lives in general.

Thromboxane A_2 increases platelet aggregation and adhesion and vasoconstriciton: prostacyclin has an opposing effect. *Aspirin* inhibits the production of TXA_2, with corresponding impairment of platelet aggregation, and it also inhibits the production of inflammatory prostaglandins.

17. Common therapeutic drugs

HYPOGLYCAEMIC AGENTS

Insulin controls carbohydrate metabolism; there may be a relative or absolute deficiency. Relative deficiency is characterized by receptor resistance. Insulin can be obtained from animal sources (pigs, cattle), but is now made by recombinant DNA technology, avoiding the risk of immune responses due to unavoidable contamination with foreign protein. It has a short half-life in plasma (5 min), and must be given frequently, in slow-release preparations or by infusion (Table 17.1).

Multiple dose and infusion regimes based on blood sugar estimations, with the aim of effecting 'tighter' control of blood glucose, are being used increasingly. This minimizes the chronic complications of hyperglycaemia viz. vascular, renal, neural and retinal complications. Perioperatively, it improves wound healing and decreases wound infection. This, however, must be balanced against the risk of undiagnosed, intraoperative hypoglycaemia.

Pharmacodynamics

1. controls the blood sugar level by promotion of glucose entry into cells
2. increases storage of glycogen in liver and muscles
3. inhibits gluconeogenesis and glycogenolysis
4. lipid production accelerated and decreased plasma lipids
5. protein synthesis is enhanced
6. lipid catabolism is inhibited, retarding ketogenesis.

Table 17.1 Insulin preparations

	Onset	Peak (hours)	Duration (hours)
Neutral insulin	30 min	2–4	6–8
Isophane insulin	3 h	6–12	18
Insulin zinc suspension (Lente)	2–3 h	7–15	24
Insulin zinc suspension crystalline (Ultralente, Ultratard)	4–6 h	10–30	24–36
Protamine zinc insulin	4–8 h	15–20	36
Biphasic insulin	30 min	4–12	24

Interactions

Corticosteroids and some diuretics (frusemide, thiazides, ethacrynic acid) lead to an increased requirement for insulin. Monoamine oxidase inhibitors and large doses of salicylates may reduce the requirement.

Oral antidiabetic agents

These may be used if the beta cells of the pancreas are still present but produce insufficient insulin.

a. **Sulphonylureas** displace insulin from the beta cells, and decrease the secretion of glucagon and liver insulinase. Tolbutamide, chlorpropamide, glibenclamide, glipizide, gliclazide and tolazamide are members of this class.

b. **Biguanide drugs.** The mode of action of this group of drugs is incompletely understood. Metformin must be used with care, particularly in patients with renal or hepatic impairment.

ANTIBIOTICS

Antibiotics impinge on anaesthetic practice as they are associated with immune responses, interact with non-depolarizing neuromuscular block, and are used in the prophylaxis of endocarditis.

Penicillin and its derivatives have a high incidence of immune reactions, from skin rashes to frank anaphylaxis. It is essential to document previous exposure to penicillin and any adverse reactions to it, and to avoid its use if there is a risk. The cephalosporin group is a suitable alternative.

Aminoglycosides (gentamicin, neomycin, streptomycin) can enhance non-depolarizing neuromuscular block which is resistant to neostigmine reversal. Prolongation of the nerve action potential by 4-amino pyridine and administration of calcium chloride have been used to promote reversal.

For the *prophylaxis of endocarditis* in patients with a past history of rheumatic heart disease, who are having dental or genitourinary procedures, or in patients with prosthetic heart valves, amoxycillin 25 mg/kg and gentamicin 2.5 mg/kg may be given on induction. If allergy to penicillin is suspected, cephazolin 20 mg/kg is substituted for amoxycillin. Cephazolin 25 mg/kg intravenously is widely used prophylactically in surgery where bacteraemia may occur; and metronidazole 7.5 mg/kg when there is a risk of anaerobic bacteraemia.

ANTICOAGULANTS

Heparin is a direct-acting anticoagulant. In low doses it slows the conversion of prothrombin to thrombin and is used in the prophylaxis of venous thrombosis. Its calcium salt is absorbed slowly after injection, maintaining an effective concentration despite the short elimination half-life of heparin (2–3 h).

In high doses it also antagonizes activated clotting factors IXa, XIa and XIIa. In doses of 300 IU/kg i.v. it abolishes clotting during cardiovascular surgery: the activated partial thromboplastin time (APPT) or activated clotting time (ACT) should be prolonged to three times control. Protamine is highly basic (in opposition to heparin which is acidic): with a dosage of 1 mg/100 IU heparin it rapidly reverses the anticoagulation. It is given slowly to avoid anaphylactoid reactions. Overdosage of protamine must be avoided as it is itself a weak anticoagulant, reducing the formation of thromboplastin.

Oral anticoagulants

Coumarins and indane diones are taken orally. They inhibit the utilization of Vitamin K, depressing the synthesis of factors, VII, IX and X and prothrombin. Their effect is delayed until these factors are depleted (this depends on the circulation t½ of the individual factors). An effect is reliably seen after 3 days. Restoration of clotting in an emergency is obtained by fresh frozen plasma and i.v. vitamin K. **Warfarin** is widely used. It is highly bound to plasma proteins. If a drug is given that competes for plasma protein (phenytoin, phenylbutazone and many others) or depresses liver metabolism (cimetidine), to a patient stabilized on a steady dose, there is a risk of overdosage. Conversely, underdosage may occur if other protein-bound drugs are stopped.

ONCOLOGICAL DRUGS

Nausea and vomiting and depressed bone marrow are common to all members of this class of drugs. Other specific system toxicities are summarized in Table 17.2.

OXYTOCICS

Oxytocic drugs stimulate the smooth muscle of the uterus to contract. These drugs are used to induce labour at term, treat postpartum atony and haemorrhage and to induce therapeutic abortion.

1. **Oxytocin.** (Syntocinon is the synthetic congener, free from the effects of vasopressin in oxytocin derived from the posterior lobe of the pituitary gland). It produces rhythmic contractions of the uterus and also facilitates lactation. Prolonged dosage may cause water intoxication, with vomiting, abdominal pain and drowsiness. Oxytocin causes a marked, but transient, vasodilator effect. This may be accompanied by reflex tachycardia. It is particularly pronounced in patients with major regional blockade, when a volatile agent is used and with large doses of oxytocin given as a bolus. Slow administration minimizes this effect.

Table 17.2 Antineoplastic drugs

Drug	Class	Major toxicity
Actinomycin D	Antibiotic	hepatic
Busulphan	Alkylating	Pulmonary fibrosis
Carmustine	Alkylating	Hepatic, pulmonary fibrosis
Chlorambucil	Alkylating	Hepatic, pulmonary fibrosis
Cisplatin	Alkylating	Renal, ototoxic, lowers Mg^{2+} and Ca^{2+}
Cyclophosphamide	Alkylating	Pulmonary fibrosis, lowers plasma cholinesterase
Cytarabine		Hepatic, neural, pulmonary
Dacarbazine	Antimetabolite	Transient liver and neural toxicity
Doxorubicin	Alkylating	Cardiomyopathy
Mercaptopurine	Antimetabolite	Hepatic necrosis
Methotrexate	Antimetabolite	Hepatic, renal and pulmonary fibrosis
Mitomycin C	Antibiotic	Renal, pulmonary infiltration
Plicamycin		Hepatic, increases bleeding, lowers Ca^{2+}, phosphate and K^+
Procarbazine		Weak MAO inhibitors
Vinblastine		Peripheral neuritis, convulsions
Vincristine		Peripheral neuritis

2. **Ergometrine** has a high affinity for alpha adrenoreceptors, directly stimulating smooth muscle. When used to control postpartum haemorrhage it should be given intramuscularly in limited dosage to avoid the risk of *hypertension*. Nausea or vomiting may follow its use. Overdosage carries the risk of gangrene of the digits.

3. **Prostaglandins.** (See Chapter 16.)

18. Dantrolene

DANTROLENE

A drug used specifically to prevent or control malignant hyperthermia during anaesthesia.

Pharmacokinetics

Oral absorption is incomplete and slow. The lyophilized powder is sparingly soluble in water: a vial contains 20 mg dantrolene sodium, 3 g mannitol and sodium hydroxide to produce a pH 9.5 when water is added. It is very irritant if given outside the veins. Plasma $t_{1/2}\beta$ is 5 h after i.v. administration. Almost all of the drug is metabolized, and excreted in urine and bile.

Pharmacodynamics

Dantrolene uncouples the excitation and contraction of skeletal muscle by interfering with Ca^{2+} release from the sarcoplasmic reticulum. Fast muscle fibres are affected more than slow ones.

Side-effects of drowsiness, dizziness and muscle weakness which occur in 20% of patients limit its value for prophylactic use.

Adverse reactions

Although these are numerous and troublesome in chronic dosage, they are very uncommon with short-term intravenous use.

Note

The sparing solubility of dantrolene (20 mg/50 ml) and the requirement of repeated dosage (1 mg/kg, repeated up to 10 mg/kg until the hyperthermia is controlled) may necessitate the administration of a large volume of water.

Azumolene is a water-soluble drug having similar actions, and is intended to overcome the problem of the large volume of solvent which has made dantrolene administration difficult.

19. Drug overdosage: principles of treatment

Deliberate self-poisoning is reported to account for 20% of admissions to an intensive care unit (ICU); 40% of patients took benzodiazepines, 31% ethyl alcohol, 12% antidepressants, 7% paracetamol. Barbiturates have been popular but now account for only 1% of admissions.

TREATMENT

1. Prevent absorption

a. Removal by inducing vomiting by oral ipecacuanha (5 ml at 6 months, 10 ml at 1 year, 15 ml at 12 years, then 30 ml) or apomorphine injection 0.07 mg/kg. (Vomiting should not be induced if protective reflexes are depressed or acids or alkalis have been taken.)

b. Adsorption to activated charcoal: reduces digoxin absorption by 40%, phenytoin by 80%, aspirin by 10%.

c. Inactivation: bicarbonate forms an insoluble salt with iron compounds.

d. Whole bowel lavage plus metoclopramide for slow release tablets (slow-K), slowly absorbed drugs and iron, lithium or mercury ingestion (e.g. in miniature batteries).

2. Increase elimination

a. Maintain renal blood flow by supporting the circulation.

b. Acidification of the urine increases pethidine excretion fivefold. It also increases excretion of tricyclic drugs, but increases their cardiovascular toxicity.

c. Haemoperfusion: passage of blood over adsorbing material.

d. Dialysis/haemofiltration. Haemodialysis is very effective for lithium and salicylates. Peritoneal dialysis is much less effective.

3. Supportive treatment

a. Cardiovascular system: maintain circulating volume and cardiac output. Inotropic drug infusions.

159

b. Respiratory system: enriched oxygen breathing or IPPV to maintain normal blood gases and acid-base.

c. Renal system: maintain urine flow with i.v. fluids and frusemide.

4. Symptomatic treatment

a. Convulsions can be controlled by i.v. thiopentone or diazepam followed by longer-acting drugs: phenytoin, phenobarbitone.

b. Cardiac arrhythmias:

    i atropine for bradycardia due to increased vagal tone

    ii beta-adrenoreceptor agonist (isoprenaline) for resistant bradycardia

    iii bicarbonate for arrhythmia caused by tricyclics.

5. Specific antidotes

a. **Naloxone** for opioid depression.

b. **Atropine** in high dosage for cholinesterase poisoning by phosphonium insecticides. A non-depolarizing neuromuscular blocker is often necessary also.

c. **N-acetylcysteine** for paracetamol overdosage. Paracetamol is a common drug in overdosage, toxicity is due to accumulation of an oxidative metabolite, N-acetyl-p-benzoquinamine. When hepatic stores of glutathione are exhausted, the metabolite binds to sulphydryl-containing protein in the liver, causing *hepatic necrosis*. N-acetylcysteine provides competing sulphydryl sites. It also carries a risk of immune reactions (rashes, bronchospasm, anaphylaxis) and may also cause hypokalaemia and interfere with platelet function.

Onset of liver damage may not be apparent for 1–2 days after ingestion: blood levels of paracetamol should be obtained as toxicity is related to its concentration and the time after ingestion.

d. **Flumazenil** is a specific antagonist of benzodiazepines, but its short plasma half-life (53 min) necessitates its repeated dosage as the half-life of benzodiazepines is much greater (diazepam t½β, 20–48 h).

e. **Pralidoxime** (2-PAM) in cholinesterase poisoning: it assists in regenerating plasma cholinesterase.

f. **Desferrioxamine** chelates iron and is excreted by the kidney and gut.

g. **Sodium bicarbonate** and **hyperventilation** for hyperkalaemia. **Insulin plus glucose** enable cells to take in K^+ during glycogen synthesis: their action is slower but lasts longer.

h. **EDTA** (calcium disodium edetate) chelates heavy metals. Cobalt EDTA removes cyanide.

i. **Hydroxocobalamin** inactivates cyanide produced in nitroprusside overdose (more than 15 $\mu g\, kg^{-1}\, min^{-1}$).

j. **Methylene blue** converts methaemoglobin back to haemoglobin. Prilocaine in doses exceeding 9 mg/kg produces clinically significant amounts of methaemoglobin.

k. **Digoxin-specific antibodies** (Fab fragments) rapidly remove digoxin from blood and bound sites (e.g. ATPase) and are rapidly excreted in urine.

20. Terminology and definitions

NAMING OF DRUGS

The *official (generic) name*, e.g. propofol, often a condensation of the *chemical name*, di-isopropyl phenol, which describes the structure.

The *brand name* is that used and patented by the manufacturer to distinguish the product: Diprivan.

DRUG DEPENDENCE

The World Health Organization definitions:

Drug abuse: persistent or sporadic excessive use inconsistent with or unrelated to acceptable medical practice.

Drug dependence: a state, psychic and sometimes also physical, resulting from the interaction between a living organism and a drug, characterized by behavioural and other responses that always include a compulsion to take the drug on a continuous or periodic basis in order to experience its psychic effects, and sometimes to avoid the discomfort of its absence. Tolerance may or may not be present. A person may be dependent on more than one drug.

DRUG DILUTIONS

1:100 000 is 0.001% or 10 μg/ml
1% is 1 g/100 ml or 10 mg/ml.

Molar solution contains 1 gram molecules/litre. For sodium bicarbonate this is 84 g/l or 8.4% (g/100 ml).

'Normal solution' in physiology is one that is isotonic with extracellular fluid: 0.9% sodium chloride, or 0.15 molar; (8.4% sodium bicarbonate is more than 6 × isotonic).

PHARMACOKINETIC TERMINOLOGY

Section 1 covers these terms: the following are repeated for quick reference.

$t_{\frac{1}{2}}\alpha$ refers to the time taken for a drug to distribute through the body and achieve its effects.

Redistribution refers to a secondary shift of drugs which are very soluble in tissues with a low perfusion: thiopentone and fat.

Volume of distribution (Vd) is a theoretical concept based on the dose of drug and the plasma concentration. It is a guide to initial dosage.

Bioavailability is the proportion of the oral dose which reaches the site of action.

$t_{1/2}\beta$ is the time taken for the plasma level to fall by 50%.

Excretion half-life is the time taken for half of the dose to appear in the urine. If a drug is partly metabolized, this figure is less informative than the plasma half-life (given above) because the effects of most drugs are related to their plasma concentrations.

Drug elimination refers to the removal of the active form of the drug by metabolism and excretion. It has replaced the term 'clearance' which has a specific physiological meaning in reference to tests of liver and renal function. The terms 'detoxication' and 'detoxification' are also obsolete as many pro-drugs are metabolized to active forms (L-dopa is metabolized in the CNS to dopamine, thyroxine is metabolized in the tissues to triiodo-thyronine). Some active drugs are metabolized to active metabolites: diazepam to oxazepam.

PHARMACODYNAMIC TERMINOLOGY

Drug effects

Therapeutic effects are those sought by the administrator: e.g paralysis by suxamethonium.

Side-effects are unwanted effects: e.g. muscle pains and twitching with suxamethonium.

Toxic effects are potentially hazardous side-effects: e.g. K^+ rise after suxamethonium (especially in burns or denervation).

Secondary effects are indirect effects: e.g. methoxyflurane is metabolized, releasing F^+. F^+ is toxic to renal tubular epithelium at plasma levels of 50 μmol/l.

Drugs and receptors

Receptors are chemical groupings on the cell membrane to which drugs become attached, then producing effects.

Acceptors are sites of attachment which do not produce effects. e.g. mucopolysaccharides and non-depolarizing neuromuscular blockers. If acceptors become saturated, further doses of the drug produce enhanced and prolonged actions.

Agonist: a drug which combines with a receptor to produce a response.

Partial agonist: a drug which combines with a receptor but does not produce a maximum response. In higher concentration partial agonists become antagonists when given with agonists.

Antagonist: a drug which combines with a receptor and blocks the effect of an agonist.

Affinity refers to the concentration of a drug which produces *50% of the maximum response.*

Intrinsic affinity: the maximum response a drug can produce (also called the *efficacy*).

Specificity refers to the effects produced by a drug at a specific receptor e.g. atropine and the muscarinic receptor.

Selectivity refers to the production of a single effect at doses less than those needed to produce all the possible effects of that drug.

Specificity and selectivity are major goals in the development of new drugs.

Effective dose (ED) has two meanings. The ED_{50} may refer to the dose which produces a response in 50% of subjects, or it may be the dose which produces 50% depression (as in neuromuscular block; more commonly ED_{95} is used in this context).

21. Clinical trials: statistics

STEPS IN DESIGNING A CLINICAL TRIAL

1. Define specifically *what is being tested*, and the *variables to be measured*, e.g:

i. for an analgesic: pain or no pain; linear analogue scale, or frequency of patient-controlled doses; total dose of drug, or several of these
ii. for an antiemetic: no vomiting, nausea, vomiting
iii. Analgesic doses: total dose of drug, or several of these
iv. for an induction agent: time of onset; pain at injection; movements; too-rapid offset, or too-prolonged action.

The questions addressed initially are the only ones which can be legitimately subjected to tests of significance on completion. The variable must be *carefully defined* e.g. duration of paralysis after neuromuscular block must define the onset (what muscle, by what test) and the offset (twitch, train-of-four, head-raising). Selection of the variable and its measurement often require expert assistance.

2. Define the *patient population* from which samples are being drawn, so that groups can be compared and variability minimized. *Results cannot be extrapolated* from the population defined.

3. Determine the *number of subjects* needed and the *type of the trial*. Assistance from the statistician is invaluable at this stage.
   Sample size (the number of subjects or trials) is determined by:

i. Variability in the population of the characteristic chosen for measurement. This may require a pilot trial.
ii. Equivalence. A true difference between the treatment–non-treatment groups is expected. A smaller difference acceptable as clinically equivalent must be defined, then the trial structured to reveal differences of greater magnitude.
iii. Avoidance of **Type I error: rejecting the null hypothesis** (see below) and accepting that the difference is significant when it is due only to biological variability.

iv. Avoidance of **Type II error: accepting the null hypothesis** when it is false, and wrongly deciding that treatment is ineffective.

The **null hypothesis** *is the assumption that there is no difference between the test and the control results. The risk of unavoidable error commonly accepted is 1 in 20 (0.05). This means that the difference reported would occur by chance only once in 20 trials. The difference is then deemed to be significant at a level of p = 0.05.*

4. Type of trial:

i. Fixed number of subjects, with analysis at completion.

ii. Sequential, with progressive assessment of results on a chart designed to reveal significance. This type of trial promotes economy of numbers, especially where large differences emerge between two treatments (see Qualitative data, below).

5. Draw samples for trial and control groups from subjects.

It is better to avoid historical controls, as retrospective selection can readily lead to error. Failure to provide any or comparable controls is repeatedly emphasized by the editors of scientific journals as the commonest error in clinical trials submitted for publication.

Avoiding bias in sampling and assessment:

i. Samples must be comparable and representative of the population being studied.

ii. Each member of the population must have an equal chance of being selected.

iii. Selected subjects must have an equal chance of entering the trial or control groups. This does not preclude pairing of subjects.

Methods:

i. Random selection and allocation, using tables of random numbers or drawing by lot.

ii. Single-, double- or triple- blind procedures, implying that the subject (single), and the administrator of the drug (double) and the observer of the results (triple) do not know which treatment is being given. Whether the subjects receive the treatment or the placebo (or other alternative) is known only to a fourth person in triple-blindness (often the pharmacist who prepares the trial drug and the 'dummy').

iii. In a drug trial the dummy or **placebo** tablets should be indistinguishable from the active drug.

6. Conduct of the trial. Specify standardization of dosages, times of administration, time and type of tests and assessments to be done, methods of recording, procedure for loss or defection of patients for any reason, and modifications made necessary by patient interests.

7. *Analysis of data* (see below).

TYPES OF DATA AND STATISTICAL ANALYSIS

The following notes are a brief overview of the principles relating to statistical analysis of experimental data. They are intended to provide a basis for discussion in the examinations and to assist in assessing articles which report experimental studies such as clinical trials. For mathematical development of the techniques reference texts should be consulted.

QUANTITATIVE DATA

Interval data

The numbers are **continuous**, representing scale units such as weight or height, so that objective measurements are comparable. If the scale starts at zero it forms a **ratio scale** where any equal interval is comparable, e.g. 20–10 equals 70–60. This type of data is frequently presented as a curve representing the 'normal distribution', the sample chosen being selected to present the 'universe'. The data are then described as being **parametric,** and the 't' test and difference of means can be applied to detect significant differences between two sets of data.

The normal distribution (See Fig. 21.1)

The curve is symmetrical (see Fig. 21.1) with equal numbers of measurements lying each side of the **mean** or average value. The mean is thus the middle value or **median**, and is also the commonest value or **mode**. 68% of observations lie within one **standard deviation** (SD) of the mean, and 95% within two SD. Hence only 5% lie in the *tails* at each end, and the probability of a value lying in one tail is thus 0.025 (2.5%). Defined features of this distribution are:

Range: the lowest to the highest value
Variance: the sum of the squared deviations from the mean divided by the number of observations
Standard deviation: the square root of the variance
Standard error of the mean: standard deviation divided by the square root of the degrees of freedom (usually one less than the number of observations).

Discrete data

Another form of quantitative data is **discrete**, measurable only in non-continuous numbers e.g. frequency of postanaesthetic vomiting. The chi-square (χ^2) test is suitable for statistical analysis of this type of data.

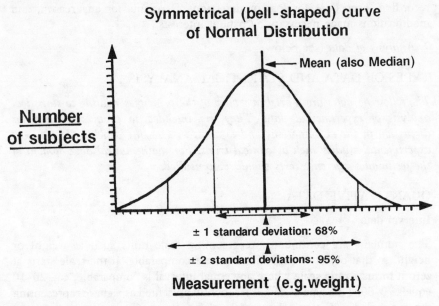

Fig. 21.1 The normal distribution. (See text for explanation.)

Analysis of variance

For two or more sets of quantitative data, the **analysis of variance (anova)** can be used to determine whether differences are due to chance.

$$\text{F-ratio} = \frac{\text{variability between treatments}}{\text{variability within treatments}}$$

Correlation coefficient

The relationship between two observations made on interval scales can also be tested by the **correlation coefficient** (see Fig. 21.2). The *line of best fit* is drawn through the observations, and the slope of this line is given by the expression:

$$y = a + bx$$

where *a* is the point where the line intersects the Y axis, and *b* is the slope of the line. The **regression coefficient, 'r'** is calculated from this slope, with values from $+1$ (positive correlation) through 0 (no correlation) to -1 (negative correlation). The curved lines giving the *95% confidence limits* can be calculated and fitted: there is a 95% probability that the plot of an observation will fall within these limits.

A *disadvantage* of correlation is that X and Y may not be causally related to one another but to a third (unspecified) variable.

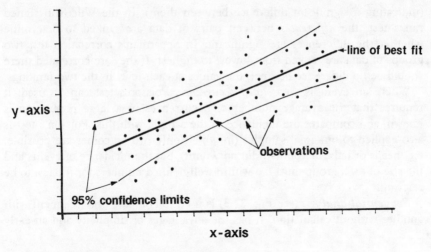

Fig. 21.2 Correlation. (See text for explanation.)

Where it is accepted that the values of Y are causally related to those of X, a regression analysis of variance can be performed, giving an F-test equivalent to the t test. The null hypothesis in this case is that the slope 'b' is zero.

QUALITATIVE DATA

1. Ordinal

Often involves subjective assessment: improved, no change, worse. The linear pain scale is ordinal even though it has numbers implying measurable intervals. Similarly the ASA anaesthetic risk scale, 1 to 5. (A common error with ordinal data is to calculate a 'mean' value e.g. add the ASA risk values together and divide by the number of patients to get an average ASA risk for a series of patients.)

2. Nominal

Mutually exclusive responses: yes/no, alive/dead.
The chi-square test is commonly used in analysis of this type of data.

OTHER TESTS

Where the test group is small and the sample can not be assumed to be representative, **non-parametric tests** are used. In the Mann–Whitney U test, the Wilcoxon sum of ranks test and the Kruskal–Wallis test the results are arranged in arithmetic order, and their position (rank) in this order used to calculate whether one group of results is higher in rank than another (indicating a significant difference between them). In the Wilcoxon signed ranks test, the *differences* between pairs of data are ranked to determine whether the differences are significant. In Spearman's correlation test two groups of data are ranked from lowest to highest. If they are correlated there should be no difference between the values at each level in the two rankings.

Where an event is an *isolated occurrence*, Poisson's test can be used: it requires that the average number of occurrences in a large population is known, and compares the incidence in the sample with this. Poisson's test is also applied to binomial samples (in which only two outcomes are possible, e.g. heads or tails, or vomited/did not vomit), but the incidence of events and the size of each group must fall within well-defined numbers for the test to be relevant.

Sequential analysis (see Fig. 21.3) is used to compare one treatment with another without calculation. It has the advantages of simplicity and an early

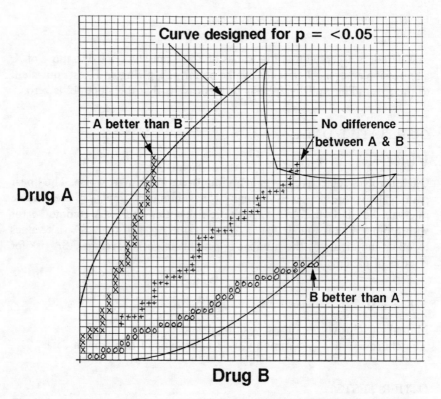

Fig. 21.3 Sequential analysis diagram. Drug A is compared with drug B; each time drug A is superior a symbol is placed in the square above the last symbol; if B is superior a symbol is placed in the square to the right; if there is no difference no symbol is entered. The sequence of x's, crossing the curve's top boundary, illustrates a trial where A was indicated to be better than B. The sequence of o's, crossing the lower boundary, show a trial where B was indicated to be better than A. The + sequence, crossing the middle boundary, indicates no difference between A and B.

end-point if there is either a large difference or no difference between the treatments.

STATISTICAL PROGRAMS

Statistical programs are now widely available, whereby the computer processes the data and prints out the results. When planning a trial it is important to seek the assistance of a statistician to ensure that:

1. the trial groups are correctly chosen
2. the observations and criteria are appropriate and non-ambiguous
3. an appropriate statistical test is applied to the data.

Computer programs do not warn the user that the data may be inappropriate for the analysis which is being proposed.

DEFINITIONS

The following definitions and explanations should be understood as they frequently arise in a discussion about trials or statistics.

Bias

The accuracy of a trial may be impaired by:

1. selecting groups which are not comparable, e.g. in age or sex
2. errors in dosage or timing
3. errors in laboratory results
4. patients dropping out, or observations being omitted
5. prejudice on the part of the patient or the observer.

Probability

When a trial has more than one possible result, this describes the chances of a particular result. The traditional example is a toss of a coin when half the outcomes will be heads and half tails. This may be expressed as 50% heads, or $p = 0.5$. (The sum of all probable outcomes is 1; if outcomes are given as percentages it is 100%.)

Probability (or 'p') is widely used in statistics because a trial can include only a sample of a population, and there is a risk that this sample is not representative. This risk is expressed as a probability. **If the risk of error is 1:20 (or 5%, or $p = 0.05$) the assumption is made in biological studies that a detected difference is significant** *(or alternatively, a lack of detected difference represents the true conclusion).*

Single- or two-tailed test

When only one end of the distribution is of interest e.g. the subjects responding to the lowest dose level of a drug, a single-tailed test may suffice.

This increases the power of an analysis as the probability value is halved (see Normal distribution).

Degrees of freedom

In a trial the degrees of freedom relate to the 'p' value tables in the statistical analysis, and are determined by the number of observations less the number of calculated parameters such as the mean. In a trial with 12 controls and 12 treated subjects, there will be two mean values (one for each group), giving $24-2 = 22$ degrees of freedom. (The assumption is that one member of each group will lie on the mean and not be 'free' to differ from it.)

Question:

Define bioavailability (or another pharmacological term). Discuss the factors affecting it.

Answer:

Define the term accurately: in this case, the amount of a drug available to the tissues as a proportion of the oral dose. The area under the plasma concentration–time curve reveals the amount available. Bioavailability is presumed to be 100% after i.v. administration.

Discussion of the factors will refer to:

1. the drug formulation and rate of absorption
2. water or lipid solubility related to absorption
3. resistance to breakdown by digestive processes
4. first-pass metabolism
5. access to tissues, e.g. blood–brain barrier.

Question:

Classify a group of drugs (*e.g. inotropes*). Compare and contrast two members (e.g. *isoprenaline with dopamine*).

Answer:

The mechanism of action would be a useful basis for classification in this case: beta-adrenoreceptor agonists, beta-adrenoreceptor modulators, adenylcyclase stimulators, phosphodiesterase inhibitors, Ca^{2+}, Na^+/K^+ ATPase inhibitors.

In comparing the two drugs, a tabular form would be appropriate, followed by a brief conclusions on the salient points of similarity and difference in relation to their clinical use.

Reference to structure–action relationships could be included in this answer.

Question:

Discuss the relevance of *some concept of pharmacology* (*e.g. pharmacogenetics*) in relation to anaesthesia.

Answer:

(*Caution must be taken to read the question carefully, and not misinterpret 'pharmacogenetics' as 'pharmacokinetics'.*)

The main discussion in this example will be on atypical plasma cholinesterases, and discussion must be accurate and the clinical consequences explained. Other topics for inclusion are malignant hyperthermia, haemoglobinopathies (susceptibility to hypoxia rather than drugs), muscular dystrophies and metabolic disorders. Immune disease and myasthenia gravis could be mentioned.

As the topic does not bear frequently on anaesthesia, an extensive knowledge would not be expected: hence the importance of a detailed knowledge of plasma cholinesterases.

In this type of question it is important to relate the discussion to anaesthesia as requested and not to digress or the answer may be seen as 'padded'.

Question:

Give an account of life-threatening reactions to drugs used in anaesthesia.

Answer:

(*Care must be taken to give a wide overview, and not confine discussion to immune responses and more obvious toxicities.*)
Suitable headings:

a. Immune responses: anaphylactic and anaphylactoid.
b. Overdosage, including relative overdosage with underlying cardiovascular, pulmonary, renal and musculoskeletal disease.
c. Genetically-based reactions – atypical plasma cholinesterase.
d. Metabolites of drugs.
e. Interactions.
f. Suxamethonium and hyperkalaemia.
g. Individual variation of response.

(Do not omit to state that respiratory or cardiovascular depression, although life-threatening, can be adequately treated when detected.)

Question:

Give an account of the pharmacology of drugs used to treat *a disease often encountered in patients presenting for anaesthesia e.g. hypertension.* (*Diabetes or asthma are also often asked, and suitable precis should be prepared.*)

Answer:

The types of action give suitable headings for the answer: in this case,

- actions on CNS
- adrenergic neurones
- adrenoreceptor blockers
- direct action on smooth muscle and cardiac muscle
- diuretics.

For each action give an example, with the mechanism of action, pharmacological principles of interest and relevant clinical applications and effect on anaesthesia including interactions.

Question

Write an account of the pharmacological basis for *some aspect of drug use in anaesthesia (e.g. premedication)*.

Answer:

Select headings which minimize the risk of repetition: it may be necessary to use specific drugs, or a drug action may be preferable with reference to the drugs which relate to it.
Suitable headings could be:

a. relief of anxiety
b. sedation
c. analgesia
d. amnesia
e. vagal block
f. antisialogogue
g. antiemetic
h. avoidance of toxicity e.g. anticonvulsant with LA
i. antacids
j. continuation of other medical treatment.

As a number of drugs fall into more than one category, it will be impossible to avoid some repetition, but it can be minimized by careful preparation of the answer.

Question:

Describe the pharmacokinetics of a *class of drugs (e.g. narcotic analgesics)*. Discuss the relevance of this information to their clinical use.

Answer:

Keep in mind that pharmacokinetics is what the body does to the drugs (pharmacodynamics refers to what the drugs do to the body). Headings will be modes of administration, absorption, distribution, metabolism and excretion. Include appropriate graphical information and equations. With this group ensure **all sites of administration are mentioned:** the absorption and distribution from epidural and subarachnoid sites will be looked for in the answer.

The second part could be discussed under headings of the various types of administration, including infusions. Each heading can conclude with a brief comment on the effectiveness of that route in achieving the goal of adequate analgesia without overdose for the desired duration, with minimal side-effects. Reference should be made to the effects of concurrent disease, age or other drugs on the kinetics of the analgesics.

Question:

Write notes on *a drug/an aspect of pharmacokinetics or pharmacodynamics/ a statistical term/a specific response (e.g. vomiting)*.

Answer:

The topic asked may sometimes be a surprise, but it is unusual not to be able either to define the term or classify the drug. As the answer is in note form, simple, brief sentences about the topic or related aspects are appropriate: a formal extensive review is not required and will take time away from that which should be allocated to other sections.

As each topic is allocated equal marks, it is possible to compensate for a weaker answer in one section by one or more sound answers in the others.

A good conclusion to each topic is a brief comment on the clinical relevance in anaesthesia.

INDEX

181

Hexafluorenium, 102
Hexamethonium in hypertension control
(use abandoned), 124
Histamine, 149, 150
Histamine$_1$ blocking drugs, 58 (Table 4.2),
59, 149–50
Histamine$_2$ blocking drugs, 46, 59, 150
Hydralazine, 26 (Table 1.3.3), 44 (Table 3.1),
125
Hydrate crystal theory of anaesthesia, 38
Hydrochlorothiazide, 134
Hydrocortisone, 147 (Table 15.1), 148
Hydrocortisone hemisuccinate, 146
Hydrolysis of drugs, 22, 23
Hydroxocobalamin in nitroprusside overdose,
127, 160
Hydroxyurea: toxic effects, 48
Hygroton *see* Chlorthalidone
Hypercalcaemia, 136 (Fig. 13.1), 137
Hypercarbia (hypercapnea), 27, 47
Hyperglycaemia, 145, 153
Hyperkalaemia, 135, 136 (Fig. 13.1), 137
treatment, 160
Hypersensitivity to drugs, 38, 41–3
tests for, 42–3
Hypertension
antihypertensive drugs, interactions, 47
treatment, 124–7
Hyperthermia, malignant, 44 (Table 3.1),
47–8, 98, 157
Hypnomidate *see* Etomidate
Hypnovel *see* Midazolam
Hypocalcaemia, 136 (Fig. 13.1), 137
Hypoglycaemic agents, 153–4
Hypokalaemia, 135, 136 (Fig. 13.1), 137,
138, 146
N-acetylcysteine as cause of, 160
digoxin toxicity relationship, 131
Hypotension
complicating drug administration, 47, 125
induced, 57, 125, 127–8

Idiosyncrasy to a drug, 38
Imipramine, 140
Immunoglobulin IgE (serum) level test for
hypersensitivity to drugs, 42
Indanediones, 155
Indapamide, 125, 134
Inderal *see* Propranolol
Indomethacin (Indocid), 70 (Table 5.5), 71
Infusion of drugs, 5–7, 69
calculation of infusion rate, 7, 21
Inhalation anaesthetics
administration, 7–9
effect on non-depolarizing blocker dosage,
106 (Table 8.6:note)
ideal characteristics of, 81–2
operating room pollution, 84

pharmacodynamics, 83
pharmacokinetics, 7–9
blood–gas equilibration, 15–17 *including*
Fig. 1.2.3 and Tables 1.2.4 & 1.2.5
minimum alveolar anaesthetic
concentration (MAC), 17 (Table
1.2.5), 83
pulmonary clearance, 16–17 *including*
Table 1.2.5
physical data, 17, 18 (Table 1.2.6)
toxicity, 82
*see also specifically named inhalation
anaesthetics*
Inorganic ions, 135–8
calcium, 136 (Fig. 13.1), 137
cardiac action relationship, 129
including Fig. 11.1, 131
muscle contraction relationship, 94, 95,
97, 98, 99, 102
lithium, 138
magnesium, 137–8
potassium, 135–7 *including* Fig. 13.1
sodium, 135
Insulin, 153–4 *including* Table 17.1
Interactions of drugs, 43–7
Class I: pharmaceutical incompatibilities,
43–4, 44
Class II: pharmacokinetic interactions, 44,
44–5
Class III: pharmacodynamic interactions,
44, 46–7
minimizing of, 48–9
Intradermal skin test for hypersensitivity to
drugs, 42
Intramuscular administration of drugs, 3–4,
69
Intrathecal administration of drugs, 9
Intravenous administration of drugs, 4–5
induction agents, 73–80
advantages of narcotic anaesthetics, 79
see also specifically named agents
Intrinsic sympathomimetic activity (ISA), 122
Ipecacuanha in drug overdosage treatment,
159
Iproniazid, 26, 46, 66
Isocarboxazid, 46, 141
Isoflurane
chemistry, 88
induced hypotension, 127
pharmacodynamics, 83, 88
pharmacokinetics, 88
blood–gas equilibration, 16 (Fig. 1.2.3)
blood–gas partition coefficient, 17
(Table 1.2.5), 88
minimum anaesthetic alveolar
concentration (MAC), 17 (Table
1.2.5), 88
oil–water partition coefficient, 17 (Table
1.2.5)

Sufentanil, 62 *including* Tables 5.1 & 5.2, 64, 79
  pharmacokinetic data, 64 (Table 5.4)
Sulphonylureas, 154
Surface application of drugs, 10–11
  sublingual, 11, 69
  see also Local anaesthetics
Surmontil *see* Trimipramine
Suxamethonium, 102, 105–7
  actions other than muscle relaxation, 47, 107–8, 137
  affinity, and attachment to receptors, 36–7
  malignant hyperthermia as complication of, 44 (Table 3.1), 47–8, 98
  metabolism, 108–9
    plasma cholinesterase relationship, 46, 99, 100 *including* Table 8.2, 108
  non-depolarizing blockers' modifying effects of, 46–7
  pregnancy, 18, 32
Synacthen, 146
Synergism in effects of drugs, 39–40 *including* Fig. 2.6
Syntocinon, 155

Tachyphylaxis, 39
Tagamet *see* Cimetidine
Tegretol *see* Carbamazepine
Temazepam, 56 *including* Table 4.1
Temgesic *see* Buprenorphine
Tenormin *see* Atenolol
Tensilon *see* Edrophonium
Terbutaline, 11, 120, 121 (Table 10.2)
Terfenadine, 149
Terminology and definitions in pharmacology, 161–3
Tetrahydroaminacrine (THA), 102
Theories of anaesthesia
  hydrate crystal theory, 38
  lipid solubility theory, 37–8
Thebaine and its derivatives, 62 (Table 5.2)
Thiazides, 126, 134, 154
  potassium loss, 46, 126
  see also specifically named thiazides
Thiethylperazine as antiemetic, 58
Thiopentone, 73, 80, 143
  intravenous injection, advantages and disadvantages, 4–5
  local anaesthetics' toxicity treatment by 116, 143
  muscle tone following administration, 94
  overdosage risk in old patients, 31
  pharmacodynamics, 75–6
  pharmacokinetics, 73–4 *including* Table 6.1
    plasma protein binding, 11–12, 73 (Table 6.1), 74
    redistribution, 14–15 *including* Fig. 1.2.2, 73

placental transfer, 18
Thioridazine, 139
Thiotepa: toxic effects of, 48
Thromboxanes
  TXA_2, 70, 151
  TXB_2, 151
Thyroxine: pro-drug nature of, 22
Tidal volume, and excretion rate, 27
Timolol (Timoptol), 120 (Table 10.1)
Tissue–blood partition coefficient, 12
Tissue perfusion, 12–15 *including* Tables 1.2.1 to 1.2.3 and Fig. 1.2.1
Tocainamide, 130
Tofranil *see* Imipramine
Tolazamide, 154
Tolazoline, 120
Tolbutamide, 154
Tolerance, 39
Torecan *see* Thiethylperazine
Tracrium *see* Atracurium
Train-of-four test for neuromuscular block, 95, 96 (Fig. 8.1), 106
Trandate *see* Labetalol
Tranquillizers, 54, 57
  hypertension control, 124
  placental transfer, 18
Tranylcypromine, 26, 46, 66, 141
Trasicor *see* Oxprenolol
Triamcinolone, 147 (Table 15.1)
Triamterene, 134
Triazolam, 56
Trichlorethylene, 17 (Table 1.2.5), 90–1
Tricyclic antidepressants, 107, 140–1
  hazards with MAOIs, 141, 142
Trifluoperazine, 139
Trimeprazine, 139, 149, 150
Trimetaphan, 128
Trimipramine, 140
Trinitrin *see* Nitroglycerine (glyceryl trinitrate)
Tryptanol *see* Amitriptyline
Tubocurarine, 39–40, 95, 104, 106 (Table 8.6)
Tyramine, 123
  monoamine oxidase inhibitor's effect on, 2, 38, 45, 141–2
Tyrosine, 123

Valium *see* Diazepam
Vallergan *see* Trimeprazine
Vasoactive drugs
  catecholamines, 119–24
    structure–action relationships, 124
  hypertension treatment, 124–7
  hypotension induced, 127–8
Vecuronium, 95, 104, 105, 106 (Table 8.6)
Ventilation–perfusion ratio (V/Q), 8, 9, 16, 27, 83
Ventolin *see* Salbutamol